Disability Psychotherapy

Disability Psychotherapy explores the growing practice of working psychotherapeutically with people with disabilities.

Over three parts, the book explores the history of disability psychotherapy, working as a disability psychotherapist and applications of disability psychotherapy. The contributors, representing a range of approaches, describe the practice of disability psychotherapy through clinical material, discuss their experiences of working in the field and reflect on their learnings. The book also considers the contributions of the Institute of Psychotherapy and Disability, and how relational attachment work with patients, colleagues, research and clinical writing creates a thriving community.

Disability Psychotherapy will be of interest to experienced and student psychotherapists, psychoanalysts, counsellors, educators, carers, parents, advocates and anyone who is concerned about widening access for people with disabilities and their networks to high quality psychotherapy treatment.

Angelina Veiga, DProf Psych Psych, is a child and adolescent psychoanalytic psychotherapist, adult psychotherapist, disability psychotherapist, clinical supervisor, researcher and visiting lecturer. A disability psychotherapist for over 20 years, she is a longstanding trustee of the Institute of Psychotherapy and Disability (IPD) and a founding member of Disability Psychotherapy Ireland.

Valerie Sinason, PhD is a poet, writer, lecturer, largely clinically retired adult psychoanalyst and President of the IPD. Having specialised in disability and trauma for 40 years, she has published or edited 25 books and over 250 papers and chapters. She was given the International Society for the Study of Trauma and Dissociation (ISSTD) Life Achievement Award in 2017 and the 2022 Innovative Excellent Award from the British Psychoanalytic Council (BPC).

'I congratulate and thank all the people who have contributed to this volume. The work has come on so far since we started the Institute of Psychotherapy and Disability and yet access to disability therapy remains poor. This book will add weight to the arguments for making disability psychotherapy available to all who need it, and as a specific training for dedicated therapists. Well done and thank you!'

Pat Frankish, *founder member, Institute of Psychotherapy and Disability; past President of the British Psychological Society*

'The authors of this wonderful book carry on the proud tradition begun by the Founders of the Institute of Psychotherapy and Disability, inspiring hope where there is often therapeutic nihilism, and understanding where there is often denial.'

Baroness Sheila Hollins, *former President of the Royal College of Psychiatry*

'Learning disabled people do have minds and can benefit cognitively and emotionally from a specialized form of psychotherapy. This is a wonderful and revelatory book.'

Anne Alvarez

Disability Psychotherapy

What It Is and Why It Matters

Edited by
Angelina Veiga and Valerie Sinason

Routledge
Taylor & Francis Group
LONDON AND NEW YORK

Designed cover image: Finn Conlon

First published 2026
by Routledge
4 Park Square, Milton Park, Abingdon, Oxon OX14 4RN

and by Routledge
605 Third Avenue, New York, NY 10158

Routledge is an imprint of the Taylor & Francis Group, an informa business

British Library Cataloguing-in-Publication Data
A catalogue record for this book is available from the British Library

ISBN: 978-1-041-08611-6 (hbk)
ISBN: 978-1-041-08609-3 (pbk)
ISBN: 978-1-003-64624-2 (ebk)

DOI: 10.4324/9781003646242

Typeset in Times New Roman
by Taylor & Francis Books

To dear friend and colleague Dr Alan Corbett, DClin.Sci, without whom this book would not have happened and whose ideas continue to inspire.

To all our contributors named and unnamed for their deep-hearted involvement in this subject and this book, especially to members of the Institute of Psychotherapy and Disability.

To our families for the love and support they provide which aids us in all we do in our life and work.

To our patients who privilege us with their rich inner core of life and never fail to surprise us.

With thanks to Sandy Dilip for her rigorous and empathic editing. She picked up this book after it had been left with multiple carers and helped us nurture it back.

And lastly our thanks to Routledge for giving this subject a voice.

Contents

Contributors

Noelle Blackman, PhD, has worked with people with learning disabilities who have experienced trauma for over 30 years. She originally trained as a Dramatherapist and is a founder member of the Institute of Psychotherapy and Disability (IPD). She is the former CEO of Respond. During her two decades at Respond she gained extensive experience in further developing the practice of psychotherapy with people with intellectual disabilities and in supporting trauma-informed practice and relational approaches in organisations. She is a regular speaker and contributor to national and international symposia and conferences. Her PhD focused on 'The Use of Psychotherapy in Supporting People with Intellectual Disabilities Who Have Experienced Bereavement'.

Elspeth Bradley, BSc, MB BS, PhD, FRCPsych, FRCPC, is a psychiatrist and psychotherapist in Intellectual Disabilities and Associate Professor at the University of Toronto, Canada. She trained in the UK (psychiatry) and Canada (psychoanalysis) and has held senior clinical and academic appointments in both countries. Her clinical practice and consulting are psychoanalytic, EMDR, polyvagal, trauma and trauma sensitive yoga informed, as well as including specific therapies and interventions. Since 2006, Elspeth has been the Mental Health Lead for the Canadian Consensus Guidelines for the Primary Care of Adults with Intellectual and Developmental Disabilities, Surrey Place (in partnership with Ontario Ministries of Health, Community and Social Services). She has published widely in peer reviewed journals and as book chapters.

Tamsin Cottis is a UKCP-registered child psychotherapist. She is a co-founder and former Assistant Director of Respond, the UK's leading provider of psychotherapeutic support to children and adults with learning disabilities. Formerly Consultant Clinical Supervisor at Respond and a teacher at the Bowlby Centre, she is a founder member of the Institute of Psychotherapy and Disability. Tamsin works as a child psychotherapist and clinical supervisor in London primary schools, in private practice and for a range of voluntary sector organisations, including Football Beyond

Borders and Young Minds. Tamsin has presented her work to a range of national and international audiences and has written widely for books and professional journals. Her most recent book is *How it Feels to be You: Objects, Play and Child Psychotherapy* (2021). Tamsin is also a published poet and prize-winning author of short stories.

Rosie Creer currently holds the role of joint Deputy Head of the Family Trauma Department at the Anna Freud Centre and is the Clinical Lead for Post Adoption. As an art psychotherapist she has 17 years' experience working with people facing multiple disadvantages and those that support them. She has held clinical management roles since 2012, supervising a wide range of clinicians, and for five years was Clinical Director at Respond. She is experienced in the development and delivery of training to professionals, and consulting to organisations, with a Diploma in Reflective Practice in Organisations from the Institute of Group Analysis. Rosie takes a trauma informed approach to her clinical work which is integrative, psychodynamic, attachment and systemic. She has extensive experience providing specialist assessment and long-term therapy to children, young people and adults, and their families who have experienced trauma; this includes developmental trauma, multiple persistent abuses, neglect and institutional harm.

Richard Curen works in private practice as a psychotherapist and supervisor and has taught and lectured across the UK and Europe. Richard is Chair of the Forensic Psychotherapy Society and is a registered member of the British Psychoanalytic Council and the British Association for Counselling and Psychotherapy. He is a board member of the International Association for Forensic Psychotherapy, a member of the Institute of Psychotherapy and Disability and a Group Analyst in Training at the Institute of Group Analysis. He is a Visiting Lecturer and Supervisor at the Portman Clinic and an Honorary Psychotherapist in the Trauma Service at the Tavistock and Portman NHS Trust. He is on the editorial board of the *International Journal for Forensic Psychotherapy* and is a reviewer for the *Journal of Intellectual Disabilities* and the *British Journal of Psychotherapy.*

Johan De Groef studied educational sciences and philosophy at KU Leuven where he is now a trainer and supervisor. He received his training as a psychoanalyst at the Belgian School of Psychoanalysis (BSP). He was the former general director of the nonprofit organization Zonnelied (Roosdaal): a residential setting and daycare centre for 200 adults with learning disabilities and severe mental health problems. He was a former chairman of the BSP and the EAMHID. He still runs a private practice as a psychoanalyst in Vilvoorde (Brussels). He has published mostly in Dutch and French. He was editor with Evelyn Heinemann of *Psychoanalysis and Mental Handicap* (1999) and with Rudi Vermote of *Verstandelijke Beperking en Psychoanalyse: Echo's van Verlangen* (2015).

Jasmine Hill, BA, MA, joined Respond in 2020 as an Art Therapist within the Midlands Transforming Care Service. Within the role Jasmine provided art therapy to children, adolescents and adults with learning disabilities, autism or both, all of whom had experienced trauma, loss and abuse. As part of Respond's Transforming Care Service, Jasmine provided relational support to people under a mental health section who were in the process of transitioning out of hospital into the community as the therapist within the individuals' circle of support. In this role she also provided the professional network with clinical thinking. In 2023, Jasmine gained a Senior Art Therapist role with Respond and took an additional position within the London Survivors Service. Jasmine has recently embarked on a new role as a CAMHS Practitioner and Art Therapist within the NHS.

Brett Kahr has worked in the mental health profession for over 40 years. At present, he serves as Senior Fellow at the Tavistock Institute of Medical Psychology in London and, also, as Visiting Professor of Psychoanalysis and Mental Health at Regent's University London. A Consultant in Psychology to The Bowlby Centre and, additionally, a Consultant Psychotherapist at The Balint Consultancy, he also holds the post of Senior Clinical Research Fellow in Psychotherapy and Mental Health at the Centre for Child Mental Health, and, additionally, the titles of Honorary Fellow and Honorary Director of Research at Freud Museum London. Professor Kahr has contributed to the media, having promoted psychotherapy and psychoanalysis in many ways, and having broadcast for many years as Resident Psychotherapist at the British Broadcasting Corporation; as a result, he then became Visiting Professor in the Faculty of Media and Communication at Bournemouth University, in recognition of his contributions. Kahr serves as Chair of the Scholars Committee of the British Psychoanalytic Council, and he is the author of eighteen books and series editor of more than eighty additional titles. His most recent books include *Bombs in the Consulting Room: Surviving Psychological Shrapnel; Dangerous Lunatics: Trauma, Criminality, and Forensic Psychotherapy; Freud's Pandemics: Surviving Global War, Spanish Flu, and the Nazis*; and *Hidden Histories of British Psychoanalysis: From Freud's Death Bed to Laing's Missing Tooth*. Professor Kahr continues to work with individuals and couples in private practice in Central London.

Jess Lammin, BA (hons), MA, has over 20 years' experience as an art psychotherapist and clinical supervisor. Jess has worked as a therapist within the NHS, charitable sector, education, forensic and CAMHS services. Her extensive experience in the field of trauma and abuse with young people led her to manage the adult survivor's psychotherapy service at Respond between 2019 and 2024 where her work with autistic people and people with learning disabilities, who had experienced trauma and abuse, consolidated her knowledge and experience. Jess went on to successfully develop and expand the service, increasing its accessibility to clients and widening its reach nationally by developing its online services during the COVID-19 pandemic.

François Marshall was born in Burgundy in 1976, to a British wine broker father and a French mother. He grew up in Paris with his older brother and mother, who resumed working as a lawyer. He met his husband Marvin in London on New Years Day 1998 when he was still studying engineering in France and moved permanently to the UK in 2000. He now lives in Kent with Marvin and works in software development. His interests include history, languages, food and travel.

Marvin Marshall-Springer was born in London in 1967 to Guianese parents. His mother worked as a nurse, whilst his father was a mechanic. Marvin grew up with his two older brothers and his younger sister. Quickly spotted at school for his singing and musical abilities, he started performing at 15. After training as a chef, he committed to a career in the music industry, working as a singer-songwriter before eventually branching out into acting. He now lives in Kent with his husband François, and still cares for James (see Chapter 13) daily. He's a keen woodworker, and loves technology and superhero movies.

Eimir McGrath, PhD, MIAHIP (Supervisor), MIAPTP (Supervisor), MIPD, ICP Reg, is a child, adolescent and adult psychotherapist who works with children, adolescents and adults. Her clinical practice focuses on complex trauma, dissociative disorders, and disability psychotherapy. Eimir is a founder member of Disability Psychotherapy Ireland and is also a committee member of the Institute of Psychotherapy and Disability (UK). She is Co-Director of Relate Ability Centre, Dublin, providing psychotherapy and clinical supervision to trainees, psychotherapists, supervisors and mental health clinicians. Eimir also delivers assessment, consultancy and training services to academic training programmes, national bodies and agencies in Ireland and Europe. Eimir is a published researcher, lecturer and trainer in several disciplines including psychotherapy, play therapy, critical disability studies, and dance; she is an invited speaker and delivers workshops at conferences both nationally and internationally in her specialist fields. Her PhD research was trans-disciplinary, combining interpersonal neurobiology, contemporary attachment theory, critical disability studies and dance.

David O'Driscoll is a leading psychoanalytic psychotherapist and historian specialising in loss, disability and bereavement for Hertfordshire Partnership University NHS Foundation Trust. This involves individual and group work with service users as well as training and consultancy to staff teams. He has had two periods as NHS Historical Worker in Hertfordshire in 2001 and as a Research Fellow at the Centre for Learning Disability Research, Hertfordshire University. He has also recently re-started the

Hertfordshire history group with Professor Bob Gates. His background prior to working in the NHS has usefully been in social work, with over 25 years of experience. From 2003–2007 David was a director of the charity Respond. He is joint convenor for the learning disability section of the Association for Psychoanalytic Psychotherapy in the National Health Service (APP) and is also a member of the Social History of the Learning Disability Research Group based at The Open University. He is also Chair and a founder member of the Institute for Psychotherapy and Disability (IPD), for whom he hosted a range of well attended and highly valued online interviews and discussions with colleagues across the Learning Disability community over the COVID-19 period. He has written papers and chapters on this work.

Georgina Parkes, MB BS MRCPsych, is a Consultant Psychiatrist in Intellectual Disability in Central and North West London NHS Foundation Trust. Previously, she worked in Hertfordshire Partnership Foundation Trust for 16 years as a Consultant Psychiatrist in Learning Disability services and has worked in the NHS since 1994. She trained as an Executive Coach with Tavistock Consulting and is registered as a senior practitioner with the European Mentoring and Coaching Council. She is a Balint group leader and was co-convener of the Association of psychoanalytic psychotherapy (APP) in the NHS, ID subgroup for many years. She is currently Treasurer for the Institute of Psychotherapy and Disability, a charity and an Honorary Senior Lecturer at Hertfordshire University in the School of Life and Medical Sciences. She has authored book chapters and papers on Gender dysphoria and ID, and Psychotherapy.

Nancy Sheppard is a Consultant Clinical Psychologist who manages a specialist Child and Adolescent Mental Health Service for children with disabilities. She has worked in the neurodevelopmental field for over 30 years. She has a particular interest in adapting psychodynamic and cognitive analytic therapeutic approaches to support emotional well-being and to build confidence in parents and carers parenting a child with additional needs. She has been a long standing member of the Institute of Psychotherapy and Disability and over her career she has played a significant role in training and supervising Clinical Psychologists, Educational Psychologists and other professionals working in this field.

Valerie Sinason, PhD, is a widely published poet, writer, lecturer, child and adolescent psychoanalytical psychotherapist (retired) and adult psychoanalyst. She has specialised in trauma and disability for 40 years and lectures nationally and internationally. She is the founder and now patron for the Clinic for Dissociative Studies UK and was also a founder member and President of the Institute for Psychotherapy and Disability. She was on the Board of the ISSTD and received their 2017 Lifetime Achievement

Award as well as the British Psychoanalytic Council Innovation Excellence award in 2022. She was an Honorary Consultant Psychotherapist at the Cape Town Child Guidance Clinic and is Chair of Trustees of the Bushman Heritage Centre, New Bethesda.

Angelina Veiga, DProf Psych Psych, is a child and adolescent psychoanalytic psychotherapist (MACP), adult psychotherapist (reg. UKCP; MICP), disability psychotherapist (MIPD), researcher, clinical supervisor, tutor and visiting lecturer. She trained at The Tavistock Centre where she taught infant and young child development and reflective practice seminars and hosted experiential groups . Angelina has worked in CAMHS, schools and specialised NHS services as a child and adolescent psychotherapist. She has also worked in several specialist trauma organisations as an adult psychotherapist. Her approach is psychoanalytically and developmentally informed. Angelina has a special interest in complex trauma, gender, disability and early childhood development. She works in private practice seeing children, adolescents, adults and families, and in the public service. She has been a trustee with the Institute of Psychotherapy and Disability for over a decade and is a founding member of Disability Psychotherapy Ireland.

Shula Wilson has been a practising psychotherapist and supervisor since 1991. She is the founder of SKYLARK (1995–2012) a charity that offered psychotherapy for people affected by disability. She is a founder member of the Institute for Psychotherapy and Disability, IPD. Shula is the author of *Counselling and Psychotherapy: Challenges and Opportunities* (2003) and has written chapters and articles on disability for various publications. Recently she edited with Ali Zarbafioth *Mother Tongue and Other Tongues* (2021).

Disability Psychotherapy

What It Is and Why It Matters

Angelina Veiga and Valerie Sinason

In 1999, psychologist, psychoanalytic psychotherapist and historian, Professor Brett Kahr had the exciting idea that a major new psycho-analytically informed disability organisation was needed. In a speedy succession of successful snowballing meetings, he raised the subject with Dr Valerie Sinason (child psychotherapist and adult psychoanalyst at St George's Hospital and the Tavistock Clinic), Baroness Sheila Hollins (psychiatrist and psychoanalytic psychotherapist), and Dr Pat Frankish (psychologist and psychoanalytic psychotherapist). He stated that the time was right in the UK for an organisation to bring together the multi-disciplinary pioneers in the field of Intellectual Disability (ID) who shared a psychoanalytic approach. Nearly 20 years of psychoanalytically informed disability therapy (from the Tavistock Clinic, St George's Hospital, Respond and the north of England) had provided the evidenced good news to share that children and adults with mild, severe and profound intellectual disability had the capacity to change through therapy. Indeed, some people with severe ID were able to transform through therapy in a way some people without ID could not! What is more, even those who could not speak could make measurable transformations through the "talking cure". We had all witnessed the changes in the lives of families and carers when meaning was explored. All of us were excited and inspired by the idea of an over-arching group as we met together regularly both formally and informally as colleagues but we needed a more formal link.

Several months later, Pat Frankish, who had also been a past President of the British Psychological Society, guided us through the application procedure so we could become a formally recognised British company. On May 20th, 2000, when Tony Blair was Prime Minister and on the same day his youngest child, Leo, was born, our group of disability pioneers held a major historical meeting at St George's Hospital at which the legendary Professor Joan Bicknell spoke, and other key members of the field attended. It cemented the beginnings of the Institute of Psychotherapy and Disability.

Six months later, on Thursday, 23rd November 2000, Dr Pat Frankish, Baroness Sheila Hollins, Dr Valerie Sinason and Prof. Brett Kahr became the four official founders of the Institute of Psychotherapy and Disability – an

DOI: 10.4324/9781003646242-1

organisation which thankfully, as Brett Kahr shows in this book (Chapter 2), continues to flourish to this day, despite the hurdles it faced and continues to face. Very quickly, a major psychological clinical and research influence in the field, Dr Nigel Beail was also invited to be a founding member. Later luminaries who joined were consultant psychiatrist Dr Roger Banks; two of the leaders of the disability charity Respond, Ms Tamsin Cottis and Dr Alan Corbett; then Dr Noelle Blackman; Dr Deborah Marks – an esteemed academic psychologist (and future child and adolescent psychotherapist); the psychiatrist Dr Georgina Parkes; David O'Driscoll; and psychotherapist Shula Wilson, who represented physical disability. They joined our community along with several others. Ultimately, at 5.00 p.m., on Monday, 18th December 2000, we held our very first meeting at the Respond headquarters, just round the corner from London's accessible Euston Station with Valerie Sinason elected as President.

The group had mainly already worked in the field for 20 years, and now, 25 years since the IPD was created, most are still working in the field, even if ostensibly retired! In other words, disability therapy has attracted an unusual group of individuals who remain faithful, passionate and deeply involved in this subject. We have listened to and read each other, supported each other and been willing to tackle the inequalities and trauma that go with this subject internally and externally.

We have been an open group, excited and appreciative of each other's work. Inspiration and learning have progressed in interesting generational lines as well as across generations. Nigel Beail was one of the examiners for the PhD's of both Pat Frankish and Valerie Sinason, whilst also being psychoanalytically influenced by them. Former supervisees of Valerie Sinason, such as Brett Kahr, Alan Corbett and Eimir McGrath also became colleagues and inspirations to her. Indeed, newer members of the IPD are themselves senior figures in the field, including David O'Driscoll, who is the very active current Chair. We have all experienced our own theories coming back to us enriched by different voices! The four key areas of the Tavistock (Sinason 1980–2000), St George's Hospital, Respond (Alan Corbett, Tamsin Cottis, Noelle Blackman, Richard Curen) and the North (Frankish and Beail) caused powerful ripples. We also had the benefit of international links, primarily, in Europe, enriched by the work of Johan De Groef and in Canada with Dr Elspeth Bradley.

Our core group were psychiatrists, psychologists, psychoanalysts and psychotherapists. Whilst coming from a range of professions the original core group had a psychoanalytic approach to disability. The Institute of Psychotherapy and Disability was originally founded to develop, accredit and regulate psychotherapists who worked with people with disabilities and aid the development of disability psychotherapy. We wished this to become an established specialism comparable to forensic psychotherapy. Our motto was "Treating with Respect" as we were concerned at the lack of access to psychological treatment for people with an intellectual disability and lack of dignity in their residential settings.

Having met with great excitement, we then addressed ourselves to our first aim. Ann Casement, as President of the UK Council of Psychotherapy (UKCP), the largest UK psychotherapy organisation, told us she wished to make disability therapy widely understood and available and once we reached 50 members we could join UKCP as a training and accrediting body. This consolidated our primary aim. By being an accrediting body, we would be able to help mainstream therapists have top-up training and increase the pool of therapists available to work with our client group.

With our small but influential team we set up a training committee and our own criteria for the number of disability cases in intensive supervised treatment, length of treatment and range of disability levels. However, when we finally reached our desired number Ann Casement was no longer President of the UKCP and we hit a brick wall. Indeed, we could see how the impact of intellectual disability had stupefied the UKCP systemic response and we had to help our membership learn that our driving aim might not be achieved. We had spent all that time and energy in order to be an accrediting body and to aid existing psychotherapists add on intellectual disability so that there would be a fairer sharing of resources with our population…it is hard to convey the level of hurt this block caused. It meant we, as professionals, were usefully experiencing in the wider professional psychotherapeutic arena, the exclusion and unwantedness our patients experienced daily.

The Jungian school within the UKCP picked up on the systemic problem of accepting intellectual disability and tried to include us. Indeed, IPD was accepted within the UKCP as a Listing Member Organisation of the Council for Psychoanalysis and Jungian Analysis. The next stage was for us to develop our accreditation criteria to reflect the broad range of therapeutic approaches represented within the current membership of the Institute. However, adjusting our aims and structures felt too complex. Whilst deciding that we needed to alter our aims and plans, Dr Pat Frankish decided to create the first Disability Psychotherapy Training through her own organisation and this has been highly successful. The change of direction from our original founding aims was cushioned by the input of Dr Angelina Veiga, child and adolescent psychoanalytic psychotherapist and adult psychotherapist; Melinda Elson and Paul Cundy; and the involvement of creative arts therapists.

In the last decade, under the Chairmanship of David O'Driscoll, there has been a vibrant underlining of our original aims with regular talks and Zooms to link us all.

We aim to provide:

- Training events targeted at clinicians seeking to work with people with disabilities.
- Collaborative work with psychotherapy, psychology and psychiatry accrediting bodies to ensure the treatment needs of people with disabilities are represented adequately in the training of clinicians.

- Development and dissemination of good practice guidelines at governmental and regional levels.
- Development and dissemination of practice-based research into the efficacy of psychotherapy with people with disabilities.
- Development of web-based resources through which psychotherapy to people with disabilities can be accessed.

We also aim:

- To provide a professional network and source of peer support.
- To advocate and lobby for psychotherapeutic treatments and approaches for people with disabilities.

However, just as the practitioners in this field are passionate and loyal, so is the shadow side of the subject. There is stigma, trauma, abuse, inequality for children and adults with ID despite the greater social understanding of their situation. There is inadequate training for many frontline staff who are also underpaid. The fear in many other professionals to come close to this subject has also not altered. This makes losses in our field even more powerful. Each IPD member is an important beating heart on our attachment map for this work.

This book was the brainchild of Dr Alan Corbett and he was to have been the editor, co-ordinator and thinker. His illness and eventual death from cancer left this book, his last active brainchild, hanging in limbo with changes in editor or co-editor due to all the complex life events that have affected people in this time of plague years. But here we are now, delighted to re-read and be re-inspired by these chapters.

Dr Alan Corbett became a therapist after social work training, a good combination for this work where the outside conditions matter so much. In 1991, he joined Tamsin Cottis at Respond, the first organisation providing psychoanalytical psychotherapy for men, women and children with learning disabilities. They worked closely with Valerie Sinason, then head of what was known as "The Mental Handicap Team" at the Tavistock Clinic in London, to help Respond's remarkable development (which was continued by Dr Noelle Blackman).

Noelle's heartfelt obituary for Alan in *Community Living* (Summer 2017) provides the key events of his professional life. In 2003 Alan returned to Ireland where he became National Director of the Child at Risk in Ireland Foundation (CARI) and made links with Dr Eimir McGrath and Dr Angelina Veiga. Coming back to England he worked as Clinical Director at Immigrant Counselling and Psychotherapy (ICAP), and as a Consultant Psychotherapist at the Clinic for Dissociative Studies, as well as in private practice, supervising work at Respond and Survivors UK, teaching at the Guild of Psychotherapists and enriching the IPD.

He completed the Portman course on Forensic Psychotherapy in 1998 and his doctorate of 2012 was published as the foundation of a solo book in 2014 – *Disabling Perversions: Forensic Psychotherapy with People with*

Intellectual Disabilities. This coincided with the time that he had his first diagnosis. He seemed eventually to recover well, continuing busily with his clinical work but sadly he became ill again.

He devoted his final months to writing, including an interview with Dr Valerie Sinason for the Festschrift he edited for her, and a major book – *Psychotherapy with Male Survivors of Sexual Abuse: The Invisible Men* (2016) which came out very shortly before he died. He was interviewed on Woman's Hour on Radio 4 (November 2016) after the launch of this book in the wake of the revelations from many young footballers that they had been sexually abused as young boys.

At a time when we all took a breath in admiration at the range of areas Alan Corbett covered and the range of skills, we lost him too quickly. His thoughtful, genuine, luminous qualities appeared in his work and relationships. We are honoured to have a chapter by two courageous men, Marvin Springer-Marshall and François Marshall, who experienced Alan as a therapist; by Dr Angelina Veiga, who experienced him as a supervisor; and indeed the co-authors of this book, who all benefitted by his kindly and rigorous eye. *Disability Psychotherapy* is the culmination of a long and painful digestion of a project that shifted shape and evolved over a protracted period of time. As an organisation we needed to make sense of the terrible loss we experienced when Alan died, and this coupled with the tremendous life changes we all underwent stalled this project. As authors many of us became identified with the experience of the disabled baby. We became in our various ways stupefied and emotionally stunted as we were without the keen eye of the loving and sensitive parent to push our development on. We needed much thinking about, vitality and care in order to pick up this project and be able to contribute to it, making it what it has evolved to be; something quite different from what Alan Corbett had envisioned. The writing of these chapters for many of us helped solidify our work as disability psychotherapists, and instilled hope and new life into an organisation that was coming out of mourning. This book has provided us the much-needed space to promote and celebrate the work we are involved in and loosen our identification with being disabled as a defence to trauma.

This important book is a book of hope. It aims to showcase how the tenets of disability psychotherapy are ingrained not only in the application of the clinical work but also as a fundamental quality within the mind of the clinician. Disabled babies need mummies and daddies in whatever shape they take, and systems that can respond, reflect and love the baby for their mere existence. These carers in turn need love and support, guidance and encouragement to claim their babies, and to work through ambivalences, disappointments, fears and hate in order to be fully present to the experience of being with their disabled child. Systems need to shift from scapegoating the most vulnerable in society to appreciating the differences in all of us, including the disabled, that enrich our experiences. The work of this book speaks of the great respect, acceptance and advocacy needed to ensure people with disabilities and their networks are helped in their everyday lives to make sense of their experiences.

The IPD faces a new dawn. Now unburdened by the monumental task of mourning and with unexpected life events now metabolised we find ourselves in a position of re-vitalisation. This book importantly contains the history, application of and struggles of disability psychotherapy. It functions to facilitate a fresh perspective to our work as disability psychotherapists, and a subtle and creative synergy has come into fruition. Now as disability psychotherapists we add inclusivity and dignity, so our patients can feel seen, heard, held and safe, as foundational aspects to our thinking. We do this by being attuned, relational and dynamic, as well as through safeguarding. It is not that we are doing anything much different than what was set out 25 years ago in those initial meetings which shaped the IPD, it is just that we are now better at describing what we do and the various ways we apply our thinking as we are less paralysed by the disabled projections and identifications we experience.

We see this book as a celebration of the work of the IPD, and of all disability psychotherapists and recipients of disability psychotherapy. We have not completed our aims of disability psychotherapy being made available to all that can benefit from it, nor have we been able to offer accreditation to all that work in this field. Instead we offer the capacity to hope, in the quiet steadiness of our work in the consulting room, with the unwavering belief that disability psychotherapy is important, matters...and that everyone should be doing it.

Angelina Veiga and Valerie Sinason
London, 2025

History of Disability Psychotherapy

Chapter 1

Implications for Training

How the Principles of Disability Psychotherapy Can Be Integrated Into Mainstream Psychotherapy Training

David O'Driscoll

In this chapter I will reflect on my experiences of becoming a 'disability psychotherapist' working in the NHS for the past 20 years and my application of the knowledge gained from this work to working as a trainer on the Bowlby Centre disability module. To my knowledge the Bowlby Centre is the only psychoanalytic psychotherapy training organization which has a module on working with people with a disability (https://thebowlbycentre.org.uk). I will also discuss my experience as a student on the D6 Tavistock course 'working psychodynamically with people with intellectual disability'. I have written in more detail on this and how this was part of my pathway to become a 'disability psychotherapist' elsewhere (O'Driscoll, 2018).

I will also discuss how I teach disability psychotherapy to psychiatrists, psychologists and trainee psychotherapists. I shall introduce and discuss the debate about mainstream or specialist services and how we can support mainstream services in meeting the obligations under the disability act for people with ID. I will then argue that the principles of 'disability psychotherapy' can help mainstream therapists, not only to work with people with ID but will help with their other clinical work too.

At the end of his long and distinguished career, the American psychiatrist Howard Potter reflected on the changes he had seen in the field of intellectual disability (ID) (Potter, 1965). Dr Potter had held many senior positions in the ID field in America and lamented the absence of psychoanalytic thinking within it. He believed that the lack of understanding of emotional difficulties such as anxiety for ID patients was due to a lack of properly trained clinicians. Potter felt this lack of insights gained from psychodynamic approaches, 'Perhaps through appropriate psychotherapeutic help and ecological manipulation the anxieties of the mental retardate can be resolved. It should be self-evident that anxiety-ridden and maladjusted mental retardates, and their number is legion, are as much entitled to psychiatric evaluation and help, as are persons who are not retardate' (Potter, 1965, 544). He believed that the problem was the pessimistic view of psychotherapeutic work with people with ID and wrote,

DOI: 10.4324/9781003646242-3

In 1920 and for a decade or more following, it was held that most of social ineffectiveness and maladjustment of the 'moron' were directly chargeable to his deficits and when emotional problems were identified in these mildly retarded subjects, these were believed to be additional man-ifestations of his constitutional inferiority. Such a hopeless concept of mental deficiency left no room for therapeutic optimism.

(Potter, 1965, 542)

Potter was rather pessimistic about his fellow professionals and wondered whether the nature of mental retardation is such that the modern psychiatrist is not so well prepared to be of service to the mentally retarded as was his nineteenth-century counterpart (Potter, 1965, 541–543). He also reported how on two previous occa-sions in 1927 and 1933, he emphasised the need for 'well-structured, dynamically oriented, professional training programs in mental deficiency' (Potter, 1965, 538). Today as I write this in May 2024, there has been no significant change. Most psychiatrists, psychologists and psychotherapists receive little if any input in work-ing psychotherapeutically with people with ID. This is despite the formation of The Institute of Psychotherapy and Disability (IPD), set up in May 2000. The IPD is a charitable body set up to promote psychotherapy for people with disabilities.

One of its aims was to promote a new breed of psychotherapist called 'disability psychotherapists', who would be specially trained and qualified to provide the 'very highest calibre of in-depth psychotherapy to these deserving individuals' (Kahr, 2000, 194). 'It is intended that it will sit alongside child psychotherapy, family therapy, forensic psychotherapy, group psychotherapy, marital psychotherapy and other such professional identities…' (Kahr, 2000, 194). The IPD has also formed a section in Ireland (2011).

Corbett (2019) has argued that we should think of this 'disability psychother-apy' as a 'transitional term'. In making this claim he is touching on one of the key debates in the field. Should there be such a specialism or should mainstream psychotherapy training include sections on working with people with ID? The IPD, which has regular conferences and training events, is currently in discus-sions with the Association for Psychoanalytic Psychotherapy in the Public Sector (APPPS) who sit within the British Psychoanalytic Council about accrediting psychotherapists to work with people via a disability section. I am hoping that this could be a forum where this debate can be pursued, drawing on the growing catalogue of literature on disability psychotherapy (see, for example, Hodges, 2003; Cottis, 2009; Jackson and Beail, 2013; Beail, 2016).

The Reason Why

There is a long list of reasons why we must find a way of overcoming what I have called 'moments of curiosity' (O'Driscoll, 2009) to creating adequate service provision for the ID community. To start with, the prevalence of mental health problems in people with ID is significantly higher than in the general population (Cooper et al., 2007). They are susceptible to the effects of loss (Blackman, 2019). They are vulnerable to abuse, trauma and bullying (i.e., Brown, Stein and Tuck, 1995; O'Driscoll, 2015). They are often likely to have additional conditions such as autism, physical disabilities, communication difficulties, self-injurious behaviour, epilepsy and life-limiting disorders. Yet, the response to these vulnerabilities has been poor. A 2015 report by Public Health England highlighted the poor care of people with ID in the British National Health Service: 'The study shows antipsychotic and antidepressant drugs are being prescribed for people with learning disabilities in England in the absence of the conditions for which they are known to be effective' (Public Health England, 2015, p. 50).

While medication has a place, there has been a long list of organisations and programmes trying to develop alternatives. The latest is NHS England with its 'Stopping Over Medication of People' (STOMP) programme. Government policies have been important in seeking to attract professional attention and resources to the needs of the ID community.

Currently there is an emphasis on client rights and client access to mainstream health services. There have been advances in human rights such as the Human Rights Act 1998 and the implementation of the Disability Discrimination Acts of 1995 and 2005. The jury is out on how successful these are. A recently published UN Report outlines the UK's failure to uphold the Convention on the Rights of People with Disabilities (2016). The report shows that, in the UK, we are still struggling to find ways of supporting disabled people to live even good enough lives and that austerity has hit people with disabilities disproportionately hard (O'Hara, 2016). Cottis (2019) has written on how these government policies were impacting on her individual psychotherapy work with children. In addition, there have been examples of high-profile scandals, such as at Winterbourne View care home (Hill, 2012). Despite all of this, the place of people with intellectual disabilities in society has changed for the better in several ways.

There are criticisms that psychological therapies do not address the underlying injustices that people face and that the emphasis should be on health promotion (Emerson and Hatton, 2014). In my view, this is not an either-or choice. I believe part of the role of 'disability therapy', may mean at times playing a more proactive role in countering injustice in people with ID lives. Marks (1999, pp. 111–112) described the therapy role as described by Sinason as a kind of 'psychoanalytic advocacy in which disability therapists, through understanding their experience, are in a privileged position to give voice to their needs'.

Therapeutic Disdain?

In the disability therapy module I teach, we consider the historical reluctance of mental health specialists to provide psychotherapy treatment for people with intellectual disabilities, starting with Sigmund Freud's (1904, p. 254) paper, 'On Psychotherapy' and his comment that, 'those patients who do not possess a reasonable degree of education and reliable character should be refused'. This early exclusion is not surprising for the period. Freud also had doubts about working with children, people with psychosis and adults over the age of 40. This exclusion, despite the early efforts of Clark and Potter, became more or less permanent so you would find comments in the classic psychoanalytic textbooks that 'mental deficiency is generally regarded as a contra-indication for psychoanalysis' (Tyson and Sandler, 1971).

The American historian, James Trent, records: 'almost all psychodynamically oriented psychiatrists saw the retarded as hardly receptive to psychodynamic insight. Indeed, most psychiatrists ... were quick to say, albeit privately, that the mentally retarded were boring' (Trent, 1994, p. 245).

This professional mindset was reinforced by cultural disdain for persons with ID. A rationale for this was provided by Francis Galton and the role of eugenics which has been so influential. Eugenics has been a dominant philosophy in the lives of people with intellectual disabilities.

If practitioners working in the field of intellectual disabilities wanted to challenge the prevailing culture by introducing a psychotherapeutic dimension to their work, there were major institutional obstacles. The clinical psychologist Seymour Sarason, considered one of the most significant American psychology researchers in education and community psychology, early in his career worked in the residential institution Southbury (in Connecticut), for people with intellectual disabilities. What struck him most was that, while the majority of his patients were from impoverished economic backgrounds, or had had brushes with the law, this was never discussed. Instead, there was a preoccupation with IQ. He noted: 'If an individual got an IQ score of 70 or above, the legal question would be asked: Have we grounds for keeping the person in the institution? There was no question about the differences between 69 and 71' (Sarason, 1988, p. 170).

While at Southbury, Sarason decided to attempt a series of 'psychotherapy studies'. He wrote:

> In those studies, I accorded them the status of persons and personhood, emphasising our similarities as thinking and feeling people and trying to counter the dominant view that they are incomplete, damaged, semi-empty vessels who are obviously human but equally obviously devoid of the 'inner life' we know so well.
>
> (Sarason, 1988, p. 157)

Sarason concluded: 'The number for whom that approach was applicable was probably not overwhelming; the psychotherapeutic endeavour is one of repair and not of prevention: and as an endeavour of repair, its results are far from perfect' (1988, pp. 157–158).

Sarason decided that this would be the best way to help patients at South-bury. If it led to a greater self-understanding by patients, or to an increase in their IQ, either way, it might help to keep the person out of institutions.

Sarason recognised that he needed professional inputs that anticipated those found in formal psychotherapy training. First, he had to have his own psychotherapy and then obtain a supervisor for his work with residents. Sarason underwent analysis with a New York psychoanalyst. 'The analysis was of enormous help to me at Southbury. For one thing, I came to understand the residents in relation to me (and vice versa) in a more complex way, both in my therapeutic work and in diagnostic work' (1988, p. 173). Sarason's appreciative comments confirm the benefits that therapists working in this field derive from having personal therapy, whether or not this leads to a full psychotherapy training. Despite Sarason seeing a prominent psychoanalyst for his personal therapy, he was turned down by other analysts for clinical supervision and then by the New York Psycho-Analytic Institute when he applied for a clinical training.

Modern Breakthrough

The critical breakthrough regarding psychoanalytic psychotherapy and ID came with the work of the psychoanalyst Neville Symington in the late 1970s and the 1980s. In his now seminal paper (Symington, 1981), he outlines the step-by-step approach to the referral of Harry. Symington was encouraged to start the psychotherapy by reading the first account of psychotherapy with people with an ID by L. Pierce Clark (1933) who had worked with Howard Potter at Letchworth Village. Symington was keen to understand why there had been minimal interest in the treatment of people with ID within the psychoanalytic community. He wrote:

'There is a strong tendency for people to despair as soon as the word organic is mentioned. Neurological growth can be stimulated and is not static. What remains static are people's expectations that change can occur' (Symington, 1981, p. 199).

Symington observed: 'There are many myths about psychotherapy and those whom it can help ... one of the myths is that a good IQ is necessary for psychotherapy to be effective. I have not witnessed such rapid change as I did in Harry in any patient of mine' (Symington, 1981, p. 198). Alongside his developing clinical work, Symington started the 'Mental Handicap Research Workshop' in 1979 at the Tavistock Clinic in London, the United Kingdom. The Tavistock remains a leading training institute for mental health professionals. At this time, the Tavistock was beginning to think about conditions not traditionally examined under the psychoanalytic lens. While Symington opened the door, the pioneering theorist was Valerie Sinason. She developed her ideas with a group of like-minded professionals from a broad section of the learning disability community. Unlike other workshops at the Tavistock clinic in this period, Sinason's meetings were open to all mental health professionals whose need for training and support was growing as long-stay hospitals were closing, and people with ID were moving into the community. I joined the Tavistock workshop in 1997 when I was struck by what a diverse group of professionals attended: psychiatrists, nurses, teachers and social workers (O'Driscoll, 2019, p 94). I remembered Sinason once telling me she saw two behavioural therapists for clinical supervision, and I queried this, 'Behavioural therapists?'.

In this field, she explained that we all shared a common concern for patients which was a key part of the philosophy underpinning the workshop and which I believe to be a key tenet underlying the philosophy of disability psychotherapy. It's motto of 'treating with respect' was fundamental. The workshop proved so popular it led to the training course, D6, which was the first course on psychodynamic approaches to people with an ID.

Responding to the needs of staff working in the field who may be interested in a psychodynamic approach, it first started as a ten-week course but developed into a year-long programme. (Sinason, 2020). It followed the established Tavistock pattern: a lecture, followed by an experiential group discussion and opportunities for participants to present material from their workplace. One of the things I found most beneficial from the course was observing a classroom in a school for children with disabilities. This component of the training was derived from the infant baby observation model and extended to the observation of other interactive settings. I was one of the last D6 cohorts before it ceased to continue. It felt like yet another missed opportunity to establish disability psychotherapy or psychotherapy-based thinking for this population. A pattern has emerged with not only psychotherapists but with organisations having 'a few moments of curiosity' (O'Driscoll, 2009) about an important subject but being unable to sustain this interest over time. This was further borne out by the IPD negotiating with the UKCP (United Kingdom Council for Psychotherapy) regarding a specialist disability section but the UKCP failing to honour this. This was followed by the setting up of the MA in psychotherapy and disability at Hertfordshire University in which I was involved. The course went via a formal procedure and was approved to be in the university prospectus. But failure to gain enough students raised the question of do workers in intellectual disabilities services want to work therapeutically with this group?

In 1996 I was working for Camden Social Services, an organisation in the vanguard of having a rights-based model for people with ID. I worked for them part-time while studying for my social work course. It was during my social work training that my curiosity about embarking upon psychotherapy training was stimulated. At the start of the training, I was unaware of the possibilities of working psychotherapeutically with this group yet I did not experience any reluctance from my training in taking on a training patient with an ID – there was a view that I should have a mixed caseload. After qualification I took on a job managing a residential service for people with ID where I was able to apply my training experiences.

Another major development was the launching of the Institute of Psychotherapy and Disability in May 2000, of which I am currently the chair. My first therapeutic post after qualifying was working as a part time loss and bereavement specialist therapist in an NHS trust. The role was established during 'the great return' (Jarrett, 2020) when long-stay hospital patients returned to the community after the institutions' closures. I worked in Hertfordshire, home to two major institutions for people with intellectual disabilities, Harperbury and Leavesden.

The Hertfordshire loss and bereavement service was set up by my colleague, Dr Noelle Blackman (Blackman, 2019). It was in response to community services noticing that despite moving to better facilities with more choice some ex-hospital patients struggled. They missed the hospital and wanted to return. Staff did not know or were unsure about the best way to support them with this loss. Helping with these and related difficulties formed the basis for my early work in the National Health Service.

Over 20 years on, my role and contribution has been viewed ambivalently, at times, perhaps reflecting the ambivalence professionals still feel about integrating persons with intellectual disabilities in the community, accepting a role for a psychodynamically informed input and a competition between rivalrous professional groups for resources in an age of austerity. I often felt my relevance in the field was questioned and felt isolated in settings where there are very few psychoanalytically oriented practitioners. There is no clear-cut career route for a psychotherapist in an intellectual disabilities service and for many years, I felt that my NHS trust did not know what to do with me.

I have written further on my personal journey as a disability psychotherapist (O'Driscoll, 2019) where I have argued that the homelessness of the disability psychotherapist reflects and parallels the unsettled status of people with intellectual disabilities in wider society. However, there is now much more of an acceptance of my place, working four days a week, running clinics where I see around twelve to fifteen service users a week. The majority are in the mid intellectual disability range.

A Clinical Example

Ms. B, who was self-harming, was cutting her arms but also cutting her hair with scissors, something that caused considerable unease and confusion for her support team. Ms. B started this behaviour following the death of her father and, after some discussion, it was established that she was not told of his death until just before the funeral, perhaps a period of a week or so. This is sadly not an uncommon response; there is often an anxiety around the person with intellectual disabilities and their reaction to grief (O'Driscoll, 2018; Blackman, 2019). I also found out that her father was a hairdresser;

both of these aspects were key elements in her self-harm. I saw her for psychotherapy, and we were able to focus on her putting into words her distress. She had a sense of being 'father's special girl' and of the betrayal and abandonment she felt. Maybe she was not so special after all.

Mainstream or Specialism?

The question of whether the mental health professions should press for the training of specialist disability psychotherapists or whether the provision of psychotherapy to clients with a disability should be provided from within mainstream mental health provision is a vitally important one for it touches on a range of issues some of which relate to the needs of specific disabilities while others relate to broader socio-political questions about the place of disabled persons within society.

There is a strong case for creating a cadre of disability psychotherapists as planned by the Institute of Psychotherapy and Disability (IPD).

Persons with intellectual disabilities can present distinctive behavioural, cognitive and emotional problems which require specialist knowledge and skills to give an adequate response.

The needs and interests of the intellectual disabilities' community are generally under-recognised and, in the past, they have been 'out of sight and out of mind'. Now more visible, as residents in the community they need more than ever the able-bodied to represent their interests and therapists who know them well are in a strong position to do this.

The Royal College of Psychiatrists did an important report into psychotherapy and people with intellectual disabilities (Beail, 2016). This report surveyed 424 responses from psychiatrists on the mailing list of the faculty of Psychiatrists of Intellectual Disability and the psychologists on the mailing list of the section of the British Psychological Society. It highlighted areas of concern:

> The particular vulnerability of this client group to sexual abuse loss psychiatric disorder consequences of institutional care was elaborated in many responses. Reference was also made to the particular problems of people with modern disabilities and personality disorders and area with clients often fall between service eligibility criteria.
>
> (Beail, 2016, pp. 28–29)

It found that 83% of respondents said there was a moderate or high demand for psychotherapy. Only three out of 424 respondents said there was no demand, and none of these worked in people with intellectual disabilities.

The evidence is that setting up disability trainings has not been easy such as with the failures of creating the UKCP disability section and the MA in Disability and Psychotherapy. The IPD is currently exploring membership links with the British Psychoanalytic Council (BPC).

But there is a counter argument.

A specialist service reinforces a medical definition of disability at a time when some voices within the disabled community are attempting to find a definition of disability which places citizenship before functional disability. Their argument is not to dismiss the significance of functional limitations but to point out that an overemphasis on them reinforces social marginalisation and social stigma. The implication of seeking to place ordinary citizenship as a defining feature of their social status leads to arguing that their psychological needs should be provided through generic mainstream services.

This argument is reinforced by two further points. Corbett argues that the therapeutic challenges presented by ID are more similar than different to the therapeutic challenges faced by other client groups. In positioning disability psychotherapy on the spectrum of therapeutic approaches, there was a temptation to focus on the differences (slower pace, often non-verbal) rather than the similarities (relational, attuned to the unconscious, transference-based) between our work and that which we tended to view as the mainstream. Moreover, he argues that seeking a specialist identity as disability therapists may be a defensive anxiety and our need for a specific label has been fed partly by our fear of danger...that our therapy is not real therapy (Corbett, 2019. p. 5).

There is the wider point that problems may present to therapists indirectly. It may be that any number of individual, couple or family problems may include the significance of a family member with an intellectual disability. In these circumstances it may be important that any therapist involved has an appreciation of what disability means and how it impacts other relatives, friends or carers. This argues for all psychotherapy training to have a module or input focused on ID. Jahoda et al point out that 'the willingness and ability of mainstream therapists to address the needs of people with intellectual disabilities remain a matter of contention' (Jahoda, Kroese and Pert, 2017, p. 246).

The evidence of mainstream services responding to the needs of the ID population is not encouraging. The IAPT (Increasing Access to Psychological Therapy) programme is an interesting case in point, set up to provide psychotherapy to the general population including people with an ID. There are many problems colleagues have encountered with it. My experience, like that of my colleague Dr Georgina Parkes, an NHS psychiatrist, has not been positive. She writes: 'In my experience, even when local intellectual disability service steps in to help facilitate these modifications, patients end up through IAPT a couple of times and then back into our specialist intellectual disability services' (Parkes, 2019, p. 82).

One wonders how seriously the IAPT is taking working with this group as a planned page on working with people with intellectual disability was still blank on their website (Jahoda, Kroese and Pert, 2017). The programme relies on people's self-referral which is clearly a barrier to our group.

The failures of the IAPT response may be due in part to the lack of good training experience leaving practitioners with anxieties and doubt. It is then inevitable that when colleagues think that a new referral is required, they will turn to a specialist intellectual disability service supported by on-going supervision or consultation with a specialist in the field to ensure continued good practice. But I believe that is not where we are at the moment, and agreed with the following by Alan Corbett in conversation with Valerie Sinason about top up training:

> I think we need both to offer 'top ups' to therapists – that's what we try to do in the IPD and through the UKCP. I think we need to be operating at the specialist level and at the barefoot level at the same time. And I think the principles we have and are there in the IPD, too, are a good fit to train workers, semi-skilled workers, and parents. Unsurprisingly though we have not been aided to disseminate it.
>
> (Corbett, 2019, p. 184)

There are therapeutic challenges to be aware of when working with people with ID, which my mainstream psychotherapy training did not prepare me for. Parsons and Upson's (1986) survey of experiences from Tavistock Clinic psychotherapists found that service users presented with behavioural challenges not encountered before in mainstream services. Psychotherapists are faced with behaviours that break the conventions of therapy. Symington (1981) wrote that these included: arriving early or late for appointments, personal questioning and inappropriate demands. Other clinicians have reported similar examples. Hodges (2003) described female service users who displayed their vagina or masturbated in sessions. Kahr (2017) discusses spitting and its challenges. This can include passivity or submissive behaviours, including the handicapped smile (Sinason, 1992) in order to placate a more powerful other. Sinason has described service users' 'awareness of death wishes' where death, damage, torture, decay, chromosomal abnormality and organic malfunction are alive in the session and the therapist has the task of facing the real hurt (Sinason, 1992, p. 81).

It is now established that the therapist needs to modify the psychoanalytic technique when working with this client group (Corbett, 2014; Jackson & Beail, 2013). Sinason (2005) addresses some of the challenges in technique. She believes that the therapist needs to work with greater flexibility and willingness to engage with the wider systems. This stands out against the idea of the psychoanalyst as a 'blank screen'. Sinason describes how the patient needs the analyst not to be the cold or abusive archaic transference figure of the survivor's history but for there to be transparency, warmth and affect. The first motto for the Institute for Psychotherapy and Disability is, 'treating with respect'. This is an acknowledgement of how historically patients with intellectual disabilities have not been treated with respect. Sinason describes the start of a psychotherapy session with a patient with intellectual disabilities in which the patient is consulted as to his wishes, thereby demonstrating the concept of 'treating with respect'. She describes this example: the therapist came to greet him at the appointment time. She said her full name, Dr Anna Alter (not her real name), and said he could call her Anna or Dr Alter and asked what would he like to be called? He was very excited and said he would like to be called Mr. Manning, Mr. Morris Manning (also a pseudonym). Dr Alter then asked Mr Manning if he would like the social worker to come in with him at the beginning to join her and the psychiatrist or whether he felt able to come by himself. Mr. Manning said he would like his social worker, Ms Worker, to come in with him for the start (Sinason, 2017, p. 16).

Disability psychotherapists often encounter limitations in the patient's ability to relate and think. This demands creativity on the therapist's side. It can be challenging and I still at times, despite my many years of practice, doubt my ability to engage with some patients. This is why supervision and being part of a supportive network is essential. It is also important to recognise what one cannot do and help our patients and their families to accept that and mourn it too.

Training

The Bowlby Centre disability module sought to help therapists in training develop the internal capacity to work with the challenges outlined above. The module is part of the institute's four-year training to be an attachment-based psychoanalytic psychotherapist. The first thing to say about the Bowlby Centre is that unlike the majority of psychotherapy training institutes, it allows their members to see patients with an ID.

The disability module was always well received and evaluated. The students found it to be a thought-provoking module and reported that it gives them the confidence to try psychotherapy with people with ID if the opportunity arrives. During my teaching time, the centre increased my input and added another seminar for the first-year students. From my point of view, as the module trainer, the key aspect I want to generate is to acknowledge their anxiety and then to develop some curiosity; that the inner life of a person with ID is interesting and worth exploring. That is why I start with history when we discuss how historically people with disabilities are on the margins of society, to understand their social exclusion, the anxiety they have generated over time, that they are 'out of mind, out of sight'.

There are several challenges to convince psychotherapists that to work with a person can have a positive therapeutic outcome; despite this, it is worth remembering what Sinason (1992) has written: 'when it comes to children and adults who are severely handicapped, professionals can sometimes shut their eyes and go stupid not just because it is painful, but because it is unbearable to see damage and not be able to repair it, not be able to put it right' (1992, p. 36).

Research has suggested that having a person with intellectual disability deliver training to the providers of services helps them to have a more positive attitude towards people (Simpson and House, 2003). In the evolution by Professor Nigel Beail of the MA into disability and psychotherapy, he commends the MA programme's use of service users' experiences as part of its teaching programme. He felt this was an admirable aspect of the course. This aspect may be something to think about for any future training.

Working with the Network

One of the key challenges for the therapist is that in most cases the therapeutic relationship is not dyadic, as the therapist is working as part of the service users' network. Working with the network is a recognised key feature of disability work (Cottis and O'Driscoll, 2009). It has been compared to child psychotherapy (Cottis, 2009) where the therapist has to consider the relationship with the child's parents. In the same way, the modern disability therapist practitioner recognises the importance of working with care staff whose cooperation is often vital. It can be a challenge: for example, Symington describes his efforts to work with his patient's support network and to enlist their assistance for the treatment. 'The staff were very willing to help. But to communicate what I had learned in a therapeutic encounter, through rational explanations, was only minimally successful' (Symington, 1981, p. 182). Staff on whom we rely to bring the service user to therapy, and to support them sympathetically may be poorly paid and relatively unsupported in their ancillary roles. They may have ambivalent and conflicting feelings, with caring and reparative feelings coexisting with feelings of anger and frustration. There may be resentment towards the therapist, who is seen as having an easy time being with the patient for just 50 minutes, rather than for up to 20 hours at a time. It is important that the person's wider network supports them having therapy and provides a containing function outside the consulting room.

Negotiating boundaries around confidentiality may be particularly difficult. Confidentiality is not always respected and support workers or family may ask intrusive questions about sessions. For these reasons, I often see the person with a member of their support network at our first meeting, where I explain what the psychotherapy involves, that I will see them every week, at the same time in the same room and that the session will last for 50 minutes in most cases, or perhaps 30 minutes. I explain that the sessions are private and confidential but that, if there is communication outside the session, I will always tell the service user. This is a difficult balancing act, as the network will have their own needs and expectations of the person in their care.

Working with family members can also be challenging. On the first meeting, I have found myself overwhelmed by relatives' psychological needs and sometimes by their difficulties in listening. The challenge of having a reciprocal conversation can seem beyond us at this point. I'm aware that the way the family presents may be the result of years of battling to get services and they may have anxiety about not being taken seriously. It also may be a moment that they are listened to by someone who does not have such a focused agenda. I always think it's important to give families space to talk and there can be tension between families and services available. Even so, we should be working towards a partnership of some description.

Working with people who have intellectual disabilities requires the same fundamental skills and values as working with any other client group:

- A non-judgmental attitude
- A non-directive approach
- Staying open to the description of a variety of experiences
- Paying attention to verbal and non-verbal information
- Awareness of transference and countertransference phenomena
- Ability to think about adaption

Who Is Afraid of Disability?

A key aspect of the course is to help students think about the impact of disability on themselves, which is difficult if we don't want to think about serious illness, impairment or disability. I start by asking the students to consider in pairs their thoughts/feelings at this moment about having a 'life-changing' disability. I show them something from a scene in *Murderball*, an award-winning documentary on athletes who are physically disabled. The scene is on how the athletes are coming to terms with disability.

We look at other accounts of disability, for example, the late Tony Judt, a writer/social historian, who had amyotrophic lateral sclerosis. Judt, wrote that

> If someone said to me five years ago, how would you feel about living in a wheelchair with a piece of Tupperware on your face all your life, I would have said no way, forget it, give me euthanasia, but in fact it's perfectly doable.
>
> (in Kane, 2019, p. 207)

I try to discuss perceptions of disability seen as 'tragic', as there is lots of evidence that their lives are seen as low quality (Kane, 2019). Able bodied people have concerns about being dependant and a feeling that they are better off dead. I also discuss the experiences of people with ID, for example, from *The Cloak of Competence*, a classic account of living with an ID after leaving a long stay hospital in America (O'Driscoll and Walmsley, 2018). One ex-hospital patient, talked of the impact of this.

> I'm real nervous and I can't always do things as good as other people, but I'd be all right if they had let me out of that institution. Anybody would

get nervous in that place. [...] I never tell people I've been in that...institution, and I always treat other people right. I talk right and I act right. I just can't seem to make people treat me like a normal person. Is it because I don't look normal?

(Edgerton, 1967, p. 170)

Today, although Freud's influence remains, especially his developing of a theory of the mind, which includes the unconscious, most therapists in this field would work from a relational perspective. It is now established that the therapist needs to modify the psychoanalytic technique when working with this client group (Corbett, 2014; Jackson & Beail, 2013).

The key way disability psychotherapy has developed is via supervision. Szecspdy (1997) highlights the Swedish term for supervision, 'handledning' which means to lead by the hand, and it is this term that most clearly shows the role supervision has had in developing disability therapy, in particularly – and almost single handedly via – Dr. Valerie Sinason, who seems to have supervised most of the key clinicians at one time or another (see Cottis, 2019). There have been many missed opportunities to establish psychotherapy beginning with Potter, Clark and Karl Menninger in the 1930s, leading to the present day. I have written elsewhere about these attempts of developing 'disability therapy', which I term 'moments of curiosity' (see O'Driscoll, 2009). One wonders what would have happened if a senior figure like Seymour Sarason had been allowed to train? For most psychotherapists, there is no formal teaching on ID or actual experience of seeing someone with an ID. And yet there is much to learn by working in a different way, and with a richly deserving group.

On reflecting on these experiences, it seems to me that the reluctance of the majority of psychotherapy training institutes to allow their members to train with patients with intellectual disability is a cruel abandonment of respect and equal opportunity, but also indicative of a primitive wish to abort people with ID from our minds.

It may be helpful to view the failure of psychotherapeutic practice to embrace fully the needs of people with intellectual disability through the lens of the 'disability transference' (Corbett, 2019). A subtle overidentification with intellectual disability may have led some of the early twentieth century pioneers to hide their work from public view, in much the same way as families have often sought to hide their learning disabled child from the glare of the community. A complex mix of shame, guilt, rage and hatred may have served to overshadow the attendant feelings of pride, joy and love that are often also present in the disability transference. A slowness, or failure, to process our transferential feelings of hatred (and love) of our patients may be seen to have been enacted in the psychotherapy community's larger disavowal of this group of patients. Our patients are 'vulnerable to psychosocial and individual perceptions of themselves as not being the "right kind of person" [...] who should have been aborted and whose own potential for procreation should be curtailed' (Corbett, 2019, p. 5).

Bibliography

Beail, N. (ed.). (2016). *Psychological Therapies and People Who Have Intellectual Disabilities.* The British Psychological Society. Commissioning team for the faculties for intellectual disabilities of the Royal College of Psychiatrists and the division of Clinical Psychology of the British Psychological Society. Leicester: The British Psychological Society.

Blackman, N. (2019). Death, loss and the struggle for non-disabled grief. In Corbett, A. (ed.), *Intellectual Disability and Psychotherapy: The Theories, Practice and Influence of Valerie Sinason* (pp. 57–70). London: Routledge.

Brown, H., Stein, J. & Tuck, V. (1995). The sexual abuse of adults with learning disabilities: Report of a second two-year incidence survey. *Mental Handicap Research* 8(1), 22–24.

Clark L. P. (1933a). The need for a better understanding of the emotional life of the feebleminded. *Proceeding Address of the American Association on Mental Deficiency*, 38, 348–357.

Clark, L. P. (1933). *The Nature and Treatment of Amentia: Psychoanalysis and Mental Arrest in Relation to the Science of Intelligence.* London: Bailliere, Tindall and Cox (American publication Baltimore, MA: William Wood and Company).

Cooper, S. A., Smiley, E., Morrison, J., Williamson, A., & Allan, L. (2007). Mental ill-health in adults with intellectual disabilities: prevalence and associated factors. *British Journal of Psychiatry*, 190, 27–35.

Corbett, A. (2014). *Disabling Perversions: Forensic Psychotherapy with People with Intellectual Disabilities.* London: Karnac Books.

Corbett, A. & Cottis, T. (2019). We are who we see looking back at us. Valerie as a supporter of a developing organisation. In Corbett, A. (ed.), *Intellectual Disability and Psychotherapy: The Theories, Practice and Influence of Valerie Sinason* (pp.34–45). London: Routledge.

Corbett, A. (ed.) (2019). *Intellectual Disability and Psychotherapy: The Theories, Practice and Influence of Valerie Sinason.* London: Routledge.

Cottis, T. (2009). *Intellectual Disability, Trauma and Psychotherapy.* London: Routledge.

Cottis, T. (2019). The disabling effects of trauma in a time of austerity: implications for the practice and theory of child psychotherapy. *Psychoanalytic Psychotherapy*, 33(3), 159–174.

Cottis, T. & O'Driscoll, D. (2009). Outside in: The effects of trauma on organisations. In Cottis, T. (2009). *Intellectual Disability, Trauma and Psychotherapy.* London: Routledge.

Edgerton, R. (1967). *The Cloak of Competence: Stigma in the Lives of the Mentally Retarded.* Berkeley, CA: University of California Press.

Emerson, E. and Hatton, C. (2014). *Heath Equalities and People with Intellectual Disabilities.* Cambridge: Cambridge University Press.

Frankish, P. (2019). Sharing our history, informing our future: Valerie Sinason and the development of training for frontline care workers and therapists. In Corbett, A. (ed.), *Intellectual Disability and Psychotherapy: The Theories, Practice and Influence of Valerie Sinason* (pp. 106–118). London: Routledge.

Frankish Training. (2017). wwwfrankishtraing.co.uk (last accessed 23 June 2021).

Freud, S. (1904). *The Complete Psychological Works of Sigmund Freud* (trans. J. Strachey), vol. 7. London: Hogarth Press.

Hill, A. (2012). Winterbourne View care home staff jailed for abusing residents. *The Guardian*, 26 October.www.theguardian.com/society/2012/oct/26/winterbourne-view-care-staff-jailed (last accessed 22 June 2021).

Hodges, S. (2003). *Counselling Adults with Learning Disabilities*. New York: Palgrave Macmillan.

Jarrett, S. (2020). *Those They Called Idiots: The Idea of the Disabled Mind from 1700 to the Present Day*. London: Reaktion Books.

Jackson, T. & Beail, N. (2013). The practice of individual psychodynamic psychotherapy with people who have intellectual disabilities. *Psychoanalytic Psychotherapy*, 27(2), 108–123.

Jahoda, A., Kroese, B. S. & Pert, C. (2017). *Cognitive Behaviour Therapy for People with Intellectual Disabilities*. London: Palgrave Macmillan.

Judt, T. (2011). *The Memory Chalet*. London: Vintage.

Kahr, B. (2000). The adventures of a psychotherapist: a new breed of clinicians – disability psychotherapists. *Psychotherapy Review*, 2, 193–194.

Kahr, B. (2017). From the treatment of a compulsive splitter: a psychoanalytical approach to profound disability. *British Journal of Psychotherapy*, 33(1), 31–47.

Kane, A. (2019). How can anyone live like that? Exploring the conscious and unconscious implications for disabled people of any chance in assisted suicide law. *British Journal of Psychotherapy*, 35(2), 195–214.

Marks, D. (1999). *Disability: Controversial Debates and Psychosocial Perspectives*. London: Routledge.

O'Driscoll, D. (2009). Psychotherapy and intellectual disability. In Cottis, T. (ed.), *Intellectual Disability, Trauma and Psychotherapy* (pp.9–28). London: Routledge.

O'Driscoll, D. (2015). Anti-hate crime. In Gates, B., Fearns, D. & Welch, J. (eds), *Learning Disability Nursing at a Glance* (p.151). Oxford: Wiley Blackwell.

O'Driscoll, D. (2019). Building insight and changing lives in intellectual disability and psychotherapy. In Corbett, A. (ed.), *Intellectual Disability and Psychotherapy: The Theories, Practice and Influence of Valerie Sinason* (pp.93–106).London: Routledge.

O'Driscoll D. (2018). Facing the final curtain. *Learning Disability Practice*, 21(3), 13.

O'Driscoll, D. & Walmsley, J. (2018). Celebrating a classic text: *The Cloak of Competence* revised. *Learning Disability Practice*, 21(5), 20.

O'Hara, J. (2016). Austerity has hit disabled people hardest – now they're fighting back. *The Guardian*, 24 February. Available at: www.theguardian.com/public-leaders-net work/2016/feb/24/austerity-disabled-people-norfolk-council-care-act (last accessed 22 November 2021).

Parkes, G. (2019). The best of both worlds: The making of a disability psychiatrist. In Corbett, A. (ed.), *Intellectual Disability and Psychotherapy: The Theories, Practice and Influence of Valerie Sinason* (pp.81–92). London: Routledge.

Parsons, J. & Upson, P. (1986). *Psychodynamic psychotherapy with mentally handicapped patients: technical issues*. Tavistock paper 3, unpublished paper.

Potter, H. W. (1965). Mental retardation: the Cinderella of psychiatry. *Psychiatry Quarterly*, 39, July, 537–549.

Sarason, S. B. (1952). Individual psychotherapy with mentally defective individuals. *American Journal of Mental Deficiency*, 56(4), 803–805.

Sarason, S. B. & Gladwin, T. (1949). *Psychological Problems in Mental Deficiency* (Third edition). New York: Harper and Brothers.

Sarason, S. B. (1988). *The Making of an American Psychologist: An Autobiography.* San Francisco, CA: Jossey Bass.

Simpson E. L. and House, A. O. (2003). User and carer involvement in mental health services: From rhetoric to science. *British Journal of Psychiatry*, 183(2), 89–91.

Sinason, V. (1992). *Mental Handicap and the Human Condition: New Approaches from the Tavistock.* London: Free Association Books.

Sinason, V. (2017). The breathing boundary. *British Journal of Psychotherapy*, 33(1), 6–16.

Sinason, V. (2020). Personal communication with author via email, May 19.

Symington, N. (1981). The psychotherapy of a subnormal patient. *British Journal of Medical Psychology*, 44, 211–228.

Szecspdy, I. (1997). Is learning possible in supervision? In Matindale, B., Morner, M. J. & Vidit J. P. (eds), *Supervision and its Vicissitudes* (pp.101–116). London: Karnac Books.

Trent, J. (1994). *Inventing the Feeble Mind: A History of Mental Retardation in America.* Berkeley, CA: University of California Press.

Turk, V. & Brown, H. (1993). The sexual abuse of adults with learning disabilities: results of a two-year incidence survey. *Mental Handicap Research*, 6, 193–216.

Tyson, R. L. & Sandler, J. (1971). Problems in the selection of patients for psychoanalysis; comments on the application of 'indications' 'suitability' and 'analysability'. *British Journal of Medical Psychology*, 44, 211–228.

Chapter 2

Three Magnificent Women and One Lovestruck Man

The Professionalism of Disability Psychotherapy

Brett Kahr

Part One

The Devastating Dismissal of Disability

Back in the late 1970s and early 1980s, as a young student of psychology, I had the privilege of attending numerous lectures and seminars on the subject of psychopathology, facilitated by some of the most esteemed academics and clinicians at several very ancient universities. Over the years, I acquired an immense degree of understanding about such conditions as schizophrenia, depression, obsessive-compulsive neuroses, criminality, anxiety, and a whole range of other diagnostic categories. But, shockingly, I do not recall a single occasion on which any of my professors or lecturers ever mentioned the word "disability" or, even, "handicap" – the traditional term used for disability during the latter decades of the twentieth century.

In those ancient days, few mental health professionals knew much, if anything, about disability, and virtually none had devoted themselves to an examination of this painfully difficult state of the mind and the body. Indeed, most psychotherapists, psychologists, psychiatrists, and psychoanalysts preferred to focus predominantly upon the more verbally lucid and well-educated patients, often those from privileged backgrounds, who might be in a better position to pay full private consultative fees.

I did not encounter a so-called "handicapped" patient until I began to work with a young man at a community mental health centre in North-West London who suffered from numerous physical illnesses and psychological infirmities, and I pleaded with my boss to permit me to explore the possibility of offering traditional psychotherapy sessions, in spite of the fact that most of my senior colleagues regarded Freudian treatment as a sheer "waste of time". Fortunately, I discovered that this person, diagnosed as "mentally handicapped", began to improve significantly as psychotherapy progressed, in spite of my youth and my relative lack of experience at that point. Consequently, I remained very committed to my work with this individual for approximately

DOI: 10.4324/9781003646242-4

ten years, during which time I continued to persevere, step by step, and, ultimately, began to provide psychoanalytical treatment to other such individuals who also suffered from a range of disabilities.

Sadly, many of my experienced psychoanalytically-informed teachers and clinical supervisors seemed surprisingly disinterested in these patients.

I shall never forget a most shocking episode. At some point during the late 1980s, while training in forensic psychotherapy at the Portman Clinic in London – an institution which specialises in the treatment of criminal offenders – I presented a case of a disabled patient, burdened by a range of both mental handicaps and physical illnesses, who had also spent time in prison for having assaulted an elderly person on the street. I had the privilege of discussing the case with a very eminent and highly experienced supervisor who had trained as both a psychiatrist and as a psychoanalyst. But, in spite of this woman's huge competence as a consultant psychiatrist, she balked, "What a disturbed patient this is, Brett. Haven't you got *a more normal patient* whom you can talk about?" It saddened me hugely that such an esteemed clinician seemed completely uninterested in my disabled client.

Fortunately, on one occasion, my professional life changed dramatically in the most unexpected and encouraging of manners.

On Saturday, 28th February 1987, I had the great opportunity to attend a special conference, hosted by the Association of Child Psychotherapists, to celebrate the 80th birthday of the iconic child psychiatrist and psychoanalyst Dr. John Bowlby. Held at the headquarters of the Zoological Society in Regent's Park, in the centre of London, this event proved extremely memorable, not least because of the very presence of the iconic Dr. Bowlby, who had the pleasure of enjoying many wonderful and much-deserved tributes delivered by numerous colleagues, including his niece, the noted child psychotherapist, Mrs. Juliet Hopkins (subsequently Dr. Hopkins). Additionally, this conference proved to be quite memorable and transformative for me, not only because of the honour of listening to those wonderful presentations but, even more so, because, at the Zoological Society, I met Mrs. Valerie Sinason for the very first time – a child psychotherapist (and subsequently an adult psychoanalyst, known as Dr. Sinason) at the Tavistock Clinic in London – who had already begun to chair that institution's Mental Handicap Psychotherapy and Psychology Research Workshop, under the auspices of the clinic's Child and Family Department.

Valerie Sinason served as one of the hosts and organisers of this special 80th-birthday tribute, and she spoke with tremendous eloquence, lucidity, and generosity about John Bowlby and his multitudinous contributions to mental health. I found her talk so riveting and so warm-hearted that, shortly after the conference, I approached her directly and asked whether she might consider offering me private clinical supervision for some of my disabled adult patients. A woman of true honourability, Sinason explained that she had not yet completed her *adult* training at that point, and, alas, she declined my request, even though she would have offered brilliant insights. At that time, she focused predominantly on children and adolescents. Nevertheless, in spite of the fact that she could not supervise my work with adults, she warmly invited me to attend regular meetings of the Mental Handicap Psychotherapy and Psychology Research Workshop, which I found tremendously helpful; and, eventually, in 1992, I delivered my very first paper on disability at the Tavistock Clinic, chaired by Sinason, entitled, "'Just Because I'm Handicapped, They Think I Don't Have a Brain': The Psycho-Analytical Psychotherapy of a Mentally Handicapped Man" (Kahr, 1992). I must confess that I felt rather intimidated to have presented my paper in front of Mrs. Sinason, who knew far more about the field of disability studies than I did; but, unsurprisingly, she responded to my presentation with her characteristic affection and encouragement, and I learned a great deal about the psychotherapeutic process by absorbing her many rich comments.

In that very same year, Valerie Sinason (1992) published her first book, the now-classic *Mental Handicap and the Human Condition: New Approaches from the Tavistock*, and I continue to maintain warm memories of the delightfully friendly launch party, held in one of the classrooms on the ground floor of the Tavistock Clinic, to honour the arrival of this terrific literary achievement. The publication of Sinason's transformative text proved so vital in many regards and certainly helped to inform us about the growing need for the psychoanalytical understanding and treatment of mentally disabled adult men, adult women, adolescents, and young children, known then, as I have indicated, as the "mentally handicapped".

As the 1990s unfolded, I enjoyed the special privilege of having become a member of the Mental Handicap Team, which Sinason co-hosted with the educational psychologist Dr. Sheila Bichard, and this experience provided me with immense instruction and encouragement in the fledgling field of offering psychoanalytically orientated treatment to those individuals suffering from severe and profound disabilities of various varieties. As my clinical experience developed, I became increasingly impressed by the ways in which these so-called "non-verbal" patients could, nevertheless, communicate extensively through facial and bodily expressions and through actions, and could, moreover, absorb our interpretative insights and benefit from our regular psychological sessions, thus enhancing a meaningful sense of attachment.

During my time at the Tavistock Clinic, I even began to work with an extremely brain-damaged, handicapped elderly woman who insisted upon lying on the couch, even though she could not speak in words; hence, through the encouragement of Sinason, Bichard, and the members of the Mental Handicap Team, I came to appreciate the ways in which classical psycho-analytical thinking and practice could, nonetheless, facilitate treatment with these non-traditional patients. This woman – a compulsive spitter – responded fantastically well to my Freudian interpretations about the potential unconscious meaning of such traumatic and destructive behaviour and, eventually, she ceased expectorating entirely, to the delight of her overburdened and exhausted nursing team and the members of her family. By having worked with this compulsive spitter, I became increasingly convinced of the benefits of traditional psychotherapy, which could, if practised intelligently, compassionately, and persistently, continue to transform these seemingly incurable individuals.

Desperate to promote the tiny, but growing, field of psychotherapeutic approaches to disability, I eventually began to lecture about the ways in which traditional psychoanalytical treatment could improve the lives of patients as frequently as possible, and, across the 1990s, I had the privilege of speaking not only to colleagues at the Tavistock Clinic (e.g., Kahr, 1993, 1994, 1995b) but, also, at a wide range of other institutions such as the British Psychological Society (Kahr, 1996), the International Association for Forensic Psychotherapy (Kahr, 1997d), and the St. Albans Counselling Centre, part of the Hertfordshire and Bedfordshire Pastoral Foundation, in the city of St. Albans (Kahr, 1998b). Additionally, I also began to develop my burgeoning skills as a writer, and, eventually, I produced a series of papers and chapters about this much-neglected subject (e.g., Kahr, 1995a, 1997a, 2017, 2020a, 2022a, 2022b, 2025).

Inspired by Valerie Sinason's growing body of impressive work (e.g., Sinason, 1986, 1988, 1990a, 1990b, 1991a, 1991b, 1993, 1994, 1996, 1998, 1999), by the encouragement of a small but valued cohort of senior colleagues at the Tavistock Clinic, and by my own growing experience as a clinician and as a lecturer, I became increasingly optimistic about the potential for improving the lives of severely and profoundly handicapped individuals and their families.

Sadly, in spite of the fact that I had the great honour to work with such pioneering leaders as Sinason, I knew only too well that few psychotherapeutic or psychoanalytical practitioners maintained any serious interest in the treatment of the disabled. Many still regarded the "disabled" as insufficiently verbally competent and, hence, incapable of free-associating in a classical Freudian manner. Thus, our disability orientated group remained, alas, rather tiny.

Clearly, we needed a bigger collegial community … and desperately so.

Part Two

A Memorable Day on the Finchley Road

Fortunately, through my participation in the Mental Handicap Team and the Mental Handicap Psychotherapy and Psychology Research Workshop (later renamed more concisely as the Mental Handicap Workshop) at the Tavistock Clinic, I began to develop not only my clinical skills, but, also, a much more public voice. In 1994, Sinason kindly appointed me as a Tutor and I began teaching disability studies to her trainees at the Tavistock Clinic.

And, in the same year, I came to meet Dr. Eileen Vizard, a hugely accomplished child psychiatrist and psychoanalyst who worked alongside Valerie

Sinason in the Child and Family Department. Vizard had studied under the iconic psychiatrist and psychoanalyst Dr. Arnon Bentovim and rapidly became one of the pioneers of child abuse studies. With great boldness, Dr. Vizard created a new service known as the Young Abusers Project – a clinical partnership between the Tavistock Clinic and the Department of Health of the United Kingdom, hosted in collaboration with the National Children's Home Action for Children, and, also, the National Society for the Prevention of Cruelty to Children – offering psychotherapeutic services to children and adolescents at risk of becoming forensic offenders. In fact, many of these young pre-criminals who had only just begun to commit their first offences (whether acts of physical violence or of sexual cruelty) suffered from disabilities as well; hence, I had the unique opportunity of joining Vizard's team, thus integrating my special interests in both forensic psychology and mental handicap (e.g., Kahr, 1997b, 2004, 2020a, 2020b, 2025).

The following year, in 1995, I became an Honorary Psychologist at St. George's Hospital in South-West London, part of the Wandsworth Community Health NHS Trust, and I enjoyed the immense honour and delight of collaborating with the hugely accomplished and forward-thinking Professor Sheila Hollins – a true pioneer of disability psychiatry, who served as head of the Division of the Psychiatry of Disability in the hospital's Department of Mental Health Sciences (e.g., Hollins, 1990a, 1990b, 1997, 2002, 2019; Hollins and Sinason, 2000). And, over the next several years, I learned a very great deal from having offered psychological assessment to Hollins's patients, diagnosed, at that time, as handicapped (Kahr, 1999).

Eventually, in 1997, after several years of having served as a lecturer for Valerie Sinason's Tavistock Clinic training programmes, namely, the D-6 course, fully titled as the "One-Year Intermediate Course on Psychodynamic Work in Mental Handicap" and later renamed as the "One-Year Intermediate Course on Psychodynamic Work in Learning Disability", and, also, the D-41 course on "Learning Disabilities and Psychotherapy", I became the Assistant Organising Tutor and, subsequently, the Chairman of the Mental Handicap Courses, part of the newly-rebranded Tavistock and Portman NHS Trust. And, in that same year, I also began to teach on several other Tavistock-based trainings, such as the Postgraduate Certificate as well as the Master of Arts course on "Child Protection: Therapeutic Approaches to Work with Children, Families and Carers Incorporating E.N.B. / C.C.E.T.S.W. 430" – the M-22 course – in which I spread our insights about the psychodynamics of disability as much as possible (e.g., Kahr, 1997e).

To my great delight, two of my former Tavistock Clinic students – Dr. Roger Banks, a Consultant Psychiatrist in Learning Disability for the North Mersey Community Trust in Liverpool, and Dr. Kathryn Lewis, a Consultant Clinical Psychologist at the Ryegate Children's Centre in Sheffield – created a small organisation in the north of England, known as the Northern Association for Psychotherapies in Learning Disability, based in Sheffield in South Yorkshire, far from the London community. I felt very proud indeed to have had the opportunity to lecture to this forward-thinking group in 1997 (Kahr, 1997c; cf. Kahr, 1998a); and, not long thereafter, I completed a short essay based on my work regarding the need for disability psychotherapy, which appeared in *The Psychotherapy Review* (Kahr, 2000a) – a journal intended for a wider group of mental health practitioners. Alas, the northern group in Sheffield did not survive for very long, but my trip to South Yorkshire certainly inspired me to consider how we might continue to develop our group of psychotherapeutically inclined practitioners more impactfully.

On Sunday morning, 9th September 1999, I cycled from my home in Hampstead, in North-West London, to the residence of Valerie Sinason, quite close by on the Finchley Road, and I arrived at 10.00 a.m. Valerie and I enjoyed a cup of coffee and a chat, and, during our conversation, I dared to propose that we might consider creating a new organisation, namely, the "Mental Handicap Institute". Despite her huge time commitments as Clinical Director of the Clinic for Dissociative Studies in London, Sinason had already devoted decades to the humanisation of disability; hence, intrigued by this idea, she endorsed my proposal and recommended that we should discuss this potential project as soon as possible with Professor Sheila Hollins. Not long thereafter, on Monday, 4th October 1999, the three of us congregated at Valerie's consulting room at 10, Harley Street, in Central London, and we began to craft a plan. Sheila endorsed the project with great enthusiasm and generosity, and, in due course, we founded "The Institute of Psychotherapy and Learning Disability", with Hollins, Kahr, and Sinason serving as the first three members of the new organisation's inaugural Executive Council.

Not long thereafter, we all agreed that it would be very helpful and very sensible to enlist the services of our dear colleague Dr. Patricia Frankish, a noted Consultant Clinical Psychologist at the Rampton Hospital in Nottinghamshire, in the north of England, who also served as Lead Psychologist for Learning Disability with the National Centre for High Secure Provision for People with Learning Disability. Frankish had, in fact, recently become elected as President of the British Psychological Society and, thus, had already proved herself as quite adept at navigating mental health organisations; moreover, like Sheila and Valerie, she, too, championed depth psychology as a form of treatment for the disabled over many years. Thus, we felt very excited to include Dr. Frankish in our burgeoning project; and, happily, round about 8.00 p.m. on Wednesday, 26th January, 2000, Pat joined us at a special meeting at Valerie's home and the four of us created the updated and revised "Institute for Psychotherapy and Disability".

Approximately thirty minutes later, at 8.30 p.m., Mrs. Ann Casement, then Chair of the United Kingdom Council for Psychotherapy, joined us for a supper, which Valerie had very kindly prepared, and helped us to consider how our newly-crafted project might collaborate with the United Kingdom's largest professional psychotherapeutic registration body. I had already enjoyed having met Mrs. Casement at a conference of the United Kingdom Council for Psychotherapy some years previously, and she had very kindly attended my Clinical Workshop on "Mental Handicap and Learning Disabilities: A Psycho-Analytical Approach" (Kahr, 1998c), part of a conference on "Development Through Diversity: Psychotherapy in Society", held at Keele University, in Keele, in the county of Staffordshire, on which occasion Casement indicated that she certainly wished to support the development of disability treatment. Happily, Mrs. Casement responded to our plans with tremendous enthusiasm and support and, ultimately, she very kindly facilitated links with this large organisation through its subdivision, namely, the College of Psychoanalysis and Jungian Analysis.

With the organisational expertise and cunning of Pat Frankish, we eventually restyled the proposed organisation, transforming the name from the "Institute for Psychotherapy and Disability" to the "Institute of Psychotherapy and Disability", and, at 8.00 p.m. on Wednesday, 10th May, 2000, the four of us held our first *official* meeting of this new organisation at Valerie's flat, once again, and became the founding Trustees.

Collectively, we crafted a mission statement, which comprised the following key points:

The Institute of Psychotherapy and Disability will endeavour to improve the quality of life of disabled citizens within the United Kingdom through setting standards for specialist training and accreditation in psychotherapy and disability.

The Institute of Psychotherapy and Disability will disseminate knowledge in the field of psychotherapy and disability.

The Institute of Psychotherapy and Disability will promote research and evaluation of the efficacy and effectiveness of psychotherapy practice.

And not long thereafter, on Saturday, 20th May 2000, Sheila Hollins kindly hosted a special launch event, chaired by her colleague Dr. Maria McGinnitty, between 10.00 a.m. and 1.00 p.m., at Hollins's long-standing institution, St. George's Hospital Medical School, part of the University of London. Happily, Sheila kindly arranged for her predecessor, the iconic psychiatrist Professor Emerita Joan Bicknell – one of the veritable founders of *disability psychiatry* (as opposed to *disability psychotherapy*) – to deliver the keynote address at this inaugural conference on "Treating with Respect". Professor Bicknell shocked us all when she reported that, not long ago, back in the 1960s, psychiatric staff would actually chain disabled in-patients to radiators as a means of both neglecting and, also, punishing these individuals (cf. Bicknell, 1994). Clearly, we had much work to undertake to ensure the greater humanisation of our patients.

Fortunately, with the support and encouragement of this devoted and accomplished group of colleagues, we all enjoyed a rich morning in the Edward Wilson Room in the Hunter Wing of St. George's Hospital Medical School, followed thereafter by a lovely lunch, and we took much pleasure that we had now formally created the new discipline of disability psychotherapy (Kahr, 2000e).

Thrilled that we had successfully launched our new organisation, I did my best to promote the Institute of Psychotherapy and Disability, and I managed to write various brief articles summarising the essence of our inaugural conference as well as our aspirations for the future (Kahr, 2000b, 2000c, 2000d).

Several months later, Pat Frankish guided us through the application procedure to become a formally recognised British company, and, on Thursday, 23rd November, 2000, Pat, Sheila, Valerie, and I became the four official founders of the Institute of Psychotherapy and Disability – an organisation which, thankfully, continues to flourish to this day. Pat kindly approached another northern-based colleague, a highly-experienced and sympathetic clinical psychologist, Dr. Nigel Beail, who also joined us as a key founding member, and, soon thereafter, other talented colleagues such as Ms. Tamsin Cottis and Mr. Alan Corbett (later Dr. Corbett) – two of the leaders of the disability charity Respond – and Dr. Deborah Marks – an esteemed academic psychologist (and future child and adolescent psychotherapist) – joined our community along with several others. Ultimately, at 5.00 p.m., on Monday, 18th December 2000, we held our very first meeting at the Respond headquarters, just round the corner from London's accessible Euston Station.

Based upon our many directorial meetings, Dr. Frankish and Dr. Beail drafted an important document, outlining the criteria for membership for our colleagues in the wider mental health profession. We agreed that for those individuals who had already qualified as psychotherapists, registered with either the British Confederation of Psychotherapists (the forerunner organisation to the British Psychoanalytic Council) or the United Kingdom Council for Psychotherapy, one must demonstrate that one will already have offered psychotherapeutic treatment to at least *ten* learning-disabled patients, at least *three* of whom will have received long-term psychotherapeutic services. And, moreover, at least *one* of the applicant's patients must have received a diagnosis of either moderate or severe learning disability. We also provided membership opportunities to other health care professionals in the learning disability field who had more recently embarked upon supervised psychotherapeutic work with such patients.

Above all, we insisted that applicants for membership must be able to demonstrate that, first and foremost, they will have treated, and will continue to treat, all disabled individuals with *respect*. Indeed, "Treating with Respect" became very much our branding catchphrase in the early days of the organisation and it remains an important philosophical bedrock to this very day.

With a team of leaders in place, and with offers of membership to our colleagues who had already demonstrated sufficient experience in the growing field of disability psychotherapy, we began to develop our fledgling organisation. In due course, we attracted over 50 registered, fee-paying members. And, thanks to the encouragement of Ann Casement, we embarked upon a dialogue with the United Kingdom Council for Psychotherapy's division known as the College of Psychoanalysis and Jungian Analysis, and I had the privilege of serving as our first representative on that board.

Before long, the Institute of Psychotherapy and Disability began to organise regular meetings and seminars in the years which unfolded, keen to spread our knowledge and to collaborate with colleagues within the field more broadly.

Part Three

From Organisational Infancy to Adulthood

As the years unfolded, our tiny organisation began to grow and to attract more attention from colleagues. We held frequent seminars and conferences, and each of us toiled hard to promote the discipline of disability psychotherapy through our clinical work, our teaching, our lecturing, and our writings. I continued to speak about the subject of disability (e.g., Kahr, 2000f), and I even managed to publish a brief article about our organisation in *The Times* newspaper (Kahr, 2005), as well as additional book chapters (e.g., Kahr, 2019, 2021). Of course, our true founder, Valerie Sinason, would produce an incomparable number of additional publications (e.g., Sinason, 2001, 2002a, 2002b, 2002c, 2002d, 2003, 2006, 2008a, 2008b, 2011a, 2011b, 2011c, 2011d, 2012, 2020, 2022a, 2022b). And many other colleagues contributed as well with rich books, compelling chapters, and interesting essays, helping to promote the field of disability psychotherapy (e.g., Beail, 1994; Corbett, Cottis, and Morris, 1996; Wilson, 1998; O'Driscoll, 1999, 2000, 2009; Blackman, 2003; Cottis, 2009a, 2009b, 2017; Corbett, 2012, 2016, 2017, 2018; Frankish, 2016; Frankish and Sinason, 2017; Corbett and Cottis, 2019; Beail, Frankish, and Skelly, 2021; Sinason and Conway, 2022), as well as the new sub-field of forensic disability psychotherapy, working with those disabled persons who also committed crimes (e.g., Curen, 2009, 2018; Corbett, 2014).

We all toiled very hard to generate interest in our organisation. And, most impressively, we gained much additional attention from the fact that our esteemed colleague Sheila Hollins ultimately became President of the Royal College of Psychiatrists in 2005 and then President of the British Medical Association in 2012, as well as a life peer in the House of Lords. In consequence, these iconic achievements and recognitions contributed much to our advancement, alongside Baroness Hollins's magnificent series of publications for disabled individuals, namely, the excellent pictorial book series entitled "Beyond Words" (e.g., Hollins and Sinason, 1992, 1993; Hollins, Horrocks, and Sinason, 2002; Sinason, Hollins, Gillani, and Laird, 2022).

Although I have sung the praises of both the Institute of Psychotherapy and Disability and of the many amazing people with whom I have had the enlightening opportunity to work over the years, not least Dr. Frankish, Baroness Hollins, and Dr. Sinason, let us recall that some brave and bold psychoanalytical practitioners had already begun to work with so-called "idiots" and so-called "cretins" and so-called "retards" during the foundational years of the psychotherapeutic profession.

Indeed, as early as 1916, Dr. Adolf Deutsch, one of the pioneering members of the *Wiener Psychoanalytische Vereinigung* [Vienna Psychoanalytical Society], supported handicapped war veterans during the *Weltkrieg* – the First World War – although we do not know fully whether he actually provided psychoanalysis as such or, rather, whether he offered general medical and physiotherapeutic assistance. Nevertheless, this overtly psychoanalytically sympathetic man certainly did devote himself to the care of this group of disabled individuals (Bronner, 2008).

And, not long thereafter, the American physician and psychoanalyst, Dr. Leon Pierce Clark (1933), contributed immensely to the field through his ground-breaking work, resulting in the publication of a little-known but, nevertheless, brilliant monograph entitled *The Nature and Treatment of Amentia: Psychoanalysis and Mental Arrest in Relation to the Science of Intelligence*, released more than 90 years ago. We might regard this title as a veritable grandparental textbook, from which we all have so much to learn.

Likewise, Dr. Simon Lindsay, a British physician and psychoanalyst, made similar contributions across the pond during the post-World War II era. Regrettably, Lindsay published virtually none of his works on the treatment of the disabled during his lifetime; but, happily, our colleague Mr. David O'Driscoll, a clinical psychotherapist and, also, a historian of psychotherapy, who ultimately became the chairperson of the Institute of Psychotherapy and Disability, managed to interview Simon Lindsay prior to the death of that distinguished psychoanalyst and has, subsequently, begun to edit Lindsay's unpublished papers. I know that we will all benefit hugely from reading this book in due course.

Other practitioners also made small, but vital, contributions to the field which became known as disability psychotherapy, such as Dr. Sándor Ferenczi (1929) from Budapest, in Hungary, and, also, Dr. Karl Menninger, from Topeka, in the American state of Kansas (Chidester and Menninger, 1936). I salute all of these iconic mental health practitioners for their incomparable work in helping us to introduce a bit more humanity into the lives of those who suffer from disabilities. I hope that by offering more therapeutic space, we, as mental health workers, will be able to ease at least a bit of the incomparable misery that burdens our planet.

Sadly, in spite of the tremendous efforts of our clinical ancestors and of our contemporaries, the Institute of Psychotherapy and Disability has still not succeeded in achieving official registration for our members through either the British Psychoanalytic Council or the United Kingdom Council for Psychotherapy. Many of our members already hold registration within these large and esteemed organisations, but not, alas, through the Institute of Psychotherapy and Disability. It may well be that some of our institutional leaders continue to maintain a slight suspicion towards, or ignorance about, the inclusion of disability. I hope that, in the years to come, this matter will eventually be resolved and that the title "disability psychotherapist" will become increasingly recognised as a more formal professional identity.

In terms of next steps, we have much more to accomplish. As for my own private hopes and fantasies for the future, I yearn for "disability psychotherapy" to become integrated as a part of every single training programme in psychology, psychiatry, counselling, social work, psychotherapy, and psychoanalysis. Moreover, I hope and trust that we will soon become recognised more officially by our national registration bodies and by many international organisations as well.

I feel very grateful to have worked alongside such amazing colleagues, all of whom comport themselves with a hugely visible sense of empathy and compassion, which often outshines the qualities of practitioners from other branches of mental health.

I salute the members of the Institute of Psychotherapy and Disability, and I hope and trust that, in due course, one of our successors will be able to write a longer and lengthier history of the achievements of this new profession in the decades and centuries to come.

Bibliography

Beail, N. (1994). "Fires, Coffins and Skeletons." In V. Sinason (Ed.). *Treating Survivors of Satanist Abuse*, pp. 153–158. London: Routledge.

Beail, N., Frankish, P., and Skelly, A. (Eds.). (2021). *Trauma and Intellectual Disability: Acknowledgement, Identification and Intervention.* Shoreham by Sea, West Sussex: Pavilion / Pavilion Publishing and Media.

Bicknell, J. (1994). Learning Disability and Ritualistic Child Abuse: Introductory Issues. In V. Sinason (Ed.). *Treating Survivors of Satanist Abuse*, pp. 151–152. London: Routledge.

Blackman, N. (2003). *Loss and Learning Disability.* London: Worth Publishing.

Bronner, A. (2008). The Members Until 1938. In A. Bronner (Ed.). *Vienna Psychoanalytic Society: The First 100 Years.* J. Morris, L. Bronner, and T. Felder (Trans.), pp. 15–74. Vienna: Christian Brandstätter Verlag.

Chidester, L., and Menninger, K. A. (1936). The Application of Psychoanalytic Methods to the Study of Mental Retardation. *American Journal of Orthopsychiatry*, 6, 616–625.

Clark, L. P. (1933). *The Nature and Treatment of Amentia: Psychoanalysis and Mental Arrest in Relation to the Science of Intelligence.* Baltimore, Maryland: William Wood and Company.

Corbett, A. (2012). Life on the Borders of Thought. In J. Adlam, A. Aiyegbusi, P. Kleinot, A. Motz, and C. Scanlon (Eds.). *The Therapeutic Milieu Under Fire: Security and Insecurity in Forensic Mental Health*, pp. 49–62. London: Jessica Kingsley Publishers.

Corbett, A. (2014). *Disabling Perversions: Forensic Psychotherapy with People with Intellectual Disabilities.* London: Karnac Books.

Corbett, A. (2016). *Psychotherapy with Male Survivors of Sexual Abuse: The Invisible Men.* London: Karnac Books.

Corbett, A. (2017). Introduction. *British Journal of Psychotherapy*, 33, 4–5.

Corbett, A. (2018). Extraordinary Therapy: On Splitting, Kindness, and Handicapping Mothers. In B. Kahr (Ed.). *New Horizons in Forensic Psychotherapy: Exploring the Work of Estela V. Welldon*, pp. 205–218. London: Karnac Books.

Corbett, A., and Cottis, T. (Eds.). (2019). *Intellectual Disability and Psychotherapy: The Theories, Practice and Influence of Valerie Sinason.* London: Routledge / Taylor and Francis Group, and Abingdon, Oxfordshire: Routledge / Taylor and Francis Group.

Corbett, A., Cottis, T., and Morris, S. (1996). *Witnessing Nurturing Protesting: Therapeutic Responses to Sexual Abuse of People with Learning Disabilities.* London: David Fulton Publishers.

Cottis, T. (Ed.). (2009a). *Intellectual Disability, Trauma and Psychotherapy.* London: Routledge / Taylor and Francis Group, and Hove, East Sussex: Routledge / Taylor and Francis Group.

Cottis, T. (2009b). Life Support or Intensive Care?: Endings and Outcomes in Psychotherapy for People with Intellectual Disabilities. In T. Cottis (Ed.). *Intellectual Disability, Trauma and Psychotherapy*, pp. 189–204. London: Routledge / Taylor and Francis Group, and Hove, East Sussex: Routledge / Taylor and Francis Group.

Cottis, T. (2017). "You *Can* Take It with You": Transitions and Transitional Objects in Psychotherapy with Children Who Have Learning Disabilities. *British Journal of Psychotherapy*, 33, 17–30.

Curen, R. (2009). "Can They See in the Door?": Issues in the Assessment and Treatment of Sex Offenders Who Have Intellectual Disabilities. In T. Cottis (Ed.). *Intellectual Disability, Trauma and Psychotherapy*, pp. 90–113. London: Routledge / Taylor and Francis Group, and Hove, East Sussex: Routledge / Taylor and Francis Group.

Curen, R. (2018). Responses to Trauma, Enactments of Trauma: The Psychodynamics of an Intellectually Disabled Family. In B. Kahr (Ed.). *New Horizons in Forensic Psychotherapy: Exploring the Work of Estela V. Welldon*, pp. 219–235. London: Karnac Books.

Ferenczi, S. (1929). The Unwelcome Child and His Death-Instinct. *International Journal of Psycho-Analysis*, 10, 125–129.

Frankish, P. (2016). *Disability Psychotherapy: An Innovative Approach to Trauma-Informed Care.* London: Karnac Books.

Frankish, P., and Sinason, V. (Eds.). (2017). *Holistic Therapy for People with Dissociative Identity Disorder.* London: Karnac Books.

Hollins, S. (1990a). Group Analytic Therapy with People with Mental Handicap. In A. Došen, A. van Gennep, and G. J. Zwanikken (Eds.). *Treatment of Mental Illness and Behavioral Disorder in the Mentally Retarded: Proceedings of the International Congress. May 3–4, 1990. Amsterdam, The Netherlands*, pp. 81–89. Leiden: Logon Publications.

Hollins, S. (1990b). Grief Therapy for People with Mental Handicap. In A. Došen, A. van Gennep, and G. J. Zwanikken (Eds.). *Treatment of Mental Illness and Behavioral Disorder in the Mentally Retarded: Proceedings of the International Congress. May 3–4, 1990. Amsterdam, The Netherlands*, pp. 139–142. Leiden: Logon Publications.

Hollins, S. (1997). Counselling and Psychotherapy. In O. Russell (Ed.). *Seminars in the Psychiatry of Learning Disabilities*, pp. 245–258. London: Gaskell / Royal College of Psychiatrists.

Hollins, S. (2002). What is the Future of the Psychiatry of Learning Disability? *Psychiatric Bulletin: The Journal of Psychiatric Practice*, 26, 283–284.

Hollins, S. (2019). Forensic Groupwork and *Books Beyond Words*: Valerie Sinason as Colleague, Co-author, and Friend. In A. Corbett and T. Cottis (Eds.). *Intellectual Disability and Psychotherapy: The Theories, Practice and Influence of Valerie*

Sinason, pp. 70–80. London: Routledge / Taylor and Francis Group, and Abingdon, Oxfordshire: Routledge / Taylor and Francis Group.

Hollins, S., Horrocks, C., and Sinason, V. (2002). *Mugged*. London: Gaskell / St. George's Hospital Medical School.

Hollins, S., and Sinason, V. (1992). *Jenny Speaks Out*. London: St George's Mental Health Library.

Hollins, S., and Sinason, V. (1993). *Bob Tells All*. London: St George's Mental Health Library.

Hollins, S., and Sinason, V. (2000). Psychotherapy, Learning Disabilities and Trauma: New Perspectives. *British Journal of Psychiatry*, 176, 32–36.

Kahr, B. (1992). *Lecture on "'Just Because I'm Handicapped, They Think I Don't Have a Brain': The Psycho-Analytical Psychotherapy of a Mentally Handicapped Man"*. Tavistock Clinic Mental Handicap Psychotherapy and Psychology Research Workshop, Child and Family Department, Tavistock Clinic, Tavistock Centre, Hampstead Health Authority, Belsize Park, London. 27th November.

Kahr, B. (1993). *Lecture on "The Treatment of a Patient with Retinitis Pigmentosa"*. Tavistock Clinic Mental Handicap Psychotherapy and Psychology Research Workshop, Child and Family Department, Tavistock Clinic, Tavistock Centre, Hampstead Health Authority, Belsize Park, London. 28th May.

Kahr, B. (1994). *Lecture on "Handicap on the Couch"*. Open Meeting, Tavistock Clinic Mental Handicap Workshop, Child and Family Department, Tavistock Clinic, Tavistock Centre, Tavistock and Portman NHS Trust, Belsize Park, London. 3rd June.

Kahr, B. (1995a). Learning Disabilities. In M. Jacobs (Ed.). *The Care Guide: A Handbook for the Caring Professions and Other Agencies*, pp. 252–261. London: Cassell.

Kahr, B. (1995b). *Lecture on "Mucus, Saliva, Urine, Faeces, Semen, Menstrual Blood, Flatus, Vomitus, and Phlegm: On Patients Who Evacuate Bodily Fluids in Psychotherapy"*. Tavistock Clinic Mental Handicap Workshop. Child and Family Department, Tavistock Clinic, Tavistock Centre, Tavistock and Portman NHS Trust, Belsize Park, London. 16th June.

Kahr, B. (1996). *Lecture on "Handicap on the Couch: The Psycho-Analytical Approach to Learning Disabilities"*. Conference on "Beyond the Basics". Special Interest Group on Learning Disabilities, Division of Clinical Psychology, British Psychological Society, Leicester, Leicestershire, at the Hill Residential College, Abergavenny, Wales. 24th April.

Kahr, B. (1997a). From the Treatment of a Compulsive Spitter: Semen, Saliva, and Alcohol Equivalents. *Intoxication, Crime and the Forensic Patient: Abstracts*, p. 10. Conference on "Intoxication, Crime and the Forensic Patient". Sixth International Conference of the International Association for Forensic Psychotherapy. Regent's College Conference Centre, Regent's College, Inner Circle, Regent's Park, London.

Kahr, B. (1997b). *Lecture on "'Plants Should Be Watered Five Days a Week': From the Psycho-Analytical Treatment of a Paedophile"*. Tuesday Evening Open Lecture / Seminar Series. Centre for Psychotherapeutic Studies, Department of Psychiatry, University of Sheffield, Sheffield, South Yorkshire. 14th January, 1997.

Kahr, B. (1997c). *Lecture on "Setting Up the Treatment: First Steps in Psychotherapy with Handicapped People"*. Conference on "Psychodynamic Approaches to Learning Disability". The Northern Association for Psychotherapies in Learning Disability, Lightwood House, Sheffield, South Yorkshire. 18th March.

Kahr, B. (1997d). *Lecture on "From the Treatment of a Compulsive Spitter: Semen, Saliva, and Alcohol Equivalents"*. Panel on Forensic Mental Handicap, Conference on "Intoxication, Crime and the Forensic Patient". Sixth International Conference, The International Association for Forensic Psychotherapy, at the Regent's College Conference Centre, Regent's College, Inner Circle, Regent's Park, London. 26th April.

Kahr, B. (1997e). *Lecture on "Mental Handicap and Child Sexual Abuse: A Case Presentation"*. Postgraduate Certificate / M.A. Degree Course on "Child Protection: Therapeutic Approaches to Work with Children, Families and Carers Incorporating E.N.B. / C.C.E.T.S.W. 430" (M-22), Child and Family Department, Tavistock Clinic, Tavistock Centre, Tavistock and Portman NHS Trust, Belsize Park, London. 26th November.

Kahr, B. (1998a). Setting Up the Treatment: First Steps in Psychotherapy with Handicapped People. In *The Association for Psychotherapies in Learning Disability (A. P.I.L.D.): Proceedings of First Conference. "Psychodynamic Approaches in Learning Disability". Sheffield. March 1997*, pp. 1–14. Sheffield, South Yorkshire: Association for Psychotherapies in Learning Disability.

Kahr, B. (1998b). *Clinical Workshop. "Handicap on the Couch: A Psychotherapeutic Approach to Mental Handicap and Learning Disabilities"*. The St. Albans Counselling Centre, Hertfordshire and Bedfordshire Pastoral Foundation, St. Albans, Hertfordshire. 10th January, 1998.

Kahr, B. (1998c). *Clinical Workshop. "Mental Handicap and Learning Disabilities: A Psycho-Analytical Approach"*. Conference on "Development Through Diversity: Psychotherapy in Society". Professional Conference, The United Kingdom Council for Psychotherapy, Keele Conference Park, Keele University, Keele, Staffordshire. 12th September, 1998.

Kahr, B. (1999). *Lecture on "The Use of the Tachistoscope in Psychodynamic Research with Mentally Handicapped Sexual Offenders"*. Developmental Disabilities Research Theme Group, Department of Psychiatry of Disability, Division of Mental Health Sciences, St. George's Hospital Medical School, University of London, Tooting, London. 24th November.

Kahr, B. (2000a). Setting Up the Treatment: First Steps in Psychotherapy with Handicapped People. *Psychotherapy Review*, 2, 536–540.

Kahr, B. (2000b). The Adventures of a Psychotherapist: A New Breed of Clinicians – Disability Psychotherapists. *Psychotherapy Review*, 2, 193–194.

Kahr, B. (2000c). The Institute of Psychotherapy and Disability. *The Psychotherapist*, 14, 18, 21.

Kahr, B. (2000d). Towards the Creation of Disability Psychotherapists. *Psychotherapy Review*, 2, 420–423.

Kahr, B. (2000e). *Lecture on "Towards the Creation of Disability Psychotherapists"*. Conference on "Treating with Respect: A Conference to Launch the Institute of Psychotherapy and Disability (A New Profession for the New Millennium)". Institute of Psychotherapy and Disability, Edward Wilson Room, Hunter Wing, St. George's Hospital Medical School, University of London, Tooting, London. 20th May.

Kahr, B. (2000f). *Lecture on "The Infanticidal Transference: Psycho-Analytical Approaches to Severe and Profound Mental Handicap"*. Post-Qualification Course VII on "Respecting Differences". Foundation for Psychotherapy and Counselling, Westminster Pastoral Foundation, London, at the London School of Economics and Political Science, University of London, London. 22nd November.

Kahr, B. (2004). Juvenile Paedophilia: The Psychodynamics of an Adolescent. In C. W. Socarides and L. R. Loeb (Eds.). *The Mind of the Paedophile: Psychoanalytic Perspectives*, pp. 95–119. London: H. Karnac (Books).

Kahr, B. (2005). Public Opinion. *Public Agenda. The Times*. 7th June, p. 3.

Kahr, B. (2017). From the Treatment of a Compulsive Spitter: A Psychoanalytical Approach to Profound Disability. *British Journal of Psychotherapy*, 33, 31–47.

Kahr, B. (2019). Valerie Sinason and the Psychodynamics of Bravery. In A. Corbett and T. Cottis (Eds.). *Intellectual Disability and Psychotherapy: The Theories, Practice and Influence of Valerie Sinason*, pp. 159–172. London: Routledge / Taylor and Francis Group, and Abingdon, Oxfordshire: Routledge / Taylor and Francis Group.

Kahr, B. (2020a). *Bombs in the Consulting Room: Surviving Psychological Shrapnel*. London: Routledge / Taylor and Francis Group, and Abingdon, Oxfordshire: Routledge / Taylor and Francis Group.

Kahr, B. (2020b). *Dangerous Lunatics: Trauma, Criminality, and Forensic Psychotherapy*. London: Confer / Confer Books.

Kahr, B. (2021). Insults and Spears: The Tribulations of Forensic Disability Psychotherapy. In N. Beail, P. Frankish, and A. Skelly (Eds.). *Trauma and Intellectual Disability: Acknowledgement, Identification and Intervention*, pp. 175–188. Shoreham by Sea, West Sussex: Pavilion / Pavilion Publishing and Media.

Kahr, B. (2022a). The Spitting Patient: Speaking with Sputum and Free-Associating with Saliva. In R. Hilty (Ed.). *Primitive Bodily Communications in Psychotherapy: Embodied Expressions of a Disembodied Psyche*, pp. 1–49, 201–207. London: Karnac / Karnac Books, Confer.

Kahr, B. (2022b). Chapter 1. In R. Hilty (Ed.). *Primitive Bodily Communications in Psychotherapy: Embodied Expressions of a Disembodied Psyche*, pp. 201–207. London: Karnac / Karnac Books, Confer.

Kahr, B. (2025). *Forensic Psychoanalysis: From Sub-Clinical Psychopaths to Serial Killers*. London: Routledge / Taylor and Francis Group, and Abingdon, Oxfordshire: Routledge / Taylor and Francis Group.

O'Driscoll, D. (1999). *A Short History of People with Learning Difficulties*. Unpublished Typescript.

O'Driscoll, D. (2000). *"The Need for a Better Understanding of the Emotional Life of the Feebleminded": Two Pioneers of Psychoanalytic Psychotherapy with People with Learning Difficulties*. M.A. in Psychotherapy and Counselling, City University, London, at the School of Psychotherapy and Counselling, Regent's College, Inner Circle, Regent's Park, London.

O'Driscoll, D. (2009). Psychotherapy and Intellectual Disability: A Historical View. In T. Cottis (Ed.). *Intellectual Disability, Trauma and Psychotherapy*, pp. 9–28. London: Routledge / Taylor and Francis Group, and Hove, East Sussex: Routledge / Taylor and Francis Group.

Sinason, V. (1986). Secondary Handicap and its Relationship to Trauma. *Psychoanalytic Psychotherapy*, 2, 131–154.

Sinason, V. (1988). Smiling, Swallowing, Sickening and Stupefying: The Effect of Sexual Abuse on the Child. *Psychoanalytic Psychotherapy*, 3, 97–111.

Sinason, V. (1990a). Individual Psychoanalytical Psychotherapy with Severely and Profoundly Handicapped Patients. In A. Došen, A. van Gennep, and G. J. Zwanikken (Eds.). *Treatment of Mental Illness and Behavioral Disorder in the Mentally*

Retarded: Proceedings of the International Congress. May 3–4, 1990. Amsterdam, The Netherlands, pp. 71–80. Leiden: Logon Publications.

Sinason, V. (1990b). Passionate Lethal Attachments. *British Journal of Psychotherapy*, 7, 66–76.

Sinason, V. (1991a). Interpretations That Feel Horrible to Make and a Theoretical Unicorn. *Journal of Child Psychotherapy*, 17, 11–24.

Sinason, V. (1991b). *A Brief and Selective Look at the History of Disability*. Unpublished Typescript.

Sinason, V. (1992). *Mental Handicap and the Human Condition: New Approaches from the Tavistock*. London: Free Association Books.

Sinason, V. (1993). *Understanding Your Handicapped Child*. London: Rosendale Press.

Sinason, V. (Ed.). (1994). *Treating Survivors of Satanist Abuse*. London: Routledge.

Sinason, V. (1996). Introduction. In A. Corbett, T. Cottis, and S. Morris. *Witnessing Nurturing Protesting: Therapeutic Responses to Sexual Abuse of People with Learning Disabilities*, pp. vii–x. London: David Fulton Publishers.

Sinason, V. (Ed.). (1998). *Memory in Dispute*. London: H. Karnac (Books).

Sinason, V. (1999). Psychoanalysis and Mental Handicap: Experience from the Tavistock Clinic. In J. De Groef and E. Heinemann (Eds.). *Psychoanalysis and Mental Handicap*. Andrew Weller (Transl.), pp. 194–206. London: Free Association Books.

Sinason, V. (2001). Children Who Kill Their Teddy Bears. In B. Kahr (Ed.). *Forensic Psychotherapy and Psychopathology: Winnicottian Perspectives*, pp. 43–49. London: H. Karnac (Books), and New York: Other Press.

Sinason, V. (Ed.). (2002a). *Attachment, Trauma and Multiplicity: Working with Dissociative Identity Disorder*. Hove, East Sussex: Brunner-Routledge / Taylor and Francis Group.

Sinason, V. (2002b). Introduction. In V. Sinason (Ed.). *Attachment, Trauma and Multiplicity: Working with Dissociative Identity Disorder*, pp. 3–20. Hove, East Sussex: Brunner-Routledge / Taylor and Francis Group.

Sinason, V. (2002c). The Shoemaker and the Elves: Working with Multiplicity. In V. Sinason (Ed.). *Attachment, Trauma and Multiplicity: Working with Dissociative Identity Disorder*, pp. 125–138. Hove, East Sussex: Brunner-Routledge / Taylor and Francis Group.

Sinason, V. (2002d). Legal Issues Around Dissociative Identity Disorder. In V. Sinason (Ed.). *Attachment, Trauma and Multiplicity: Working with Dissociative Identity Disorder*, pp. 206–207. Hove, East Sussex: Brunner-Routledge / Taylor and Francis Group.

Sinason, V. (2003). Foreword. In N. Blackman. *Loss and Learning Disability*, pp. xi–xii. London: Worth Publishing.

Sinason, V. (2006). No Touch Please – We're British Psychodynamic Practitioners. In G. Galton (Ed.). *Touch Papers: Dialogues on Touch in the Psychoanalytic Space*, pp. 49–60. London: Karnac Books.

Sinason, V. (2008a). Finding Abused Children's Voices: Junior-School Living Nightmares. In R. Campher (Ed.). *Violence in Children: Understanding and Helping Those Who Harm*, pp. 211–227. London: Karnac Books.

Sinason, V. (2008b). When Murder Moves Inside. In A. Sachs and G. Galton (Eds.). *Forensic Aspects of Dissociative Identity Disorder*, pp. 100–107. London: Karnac Books.

Sinason, V. (Ed.). (2011a). *Attachment, Trauma and Multiplicity: Second Edition. Working with Dissociative Identity Disorder*. London: Routledge / Taylor and Francis Group, and Hove, East Sussex: Routledge / Taylor and Francis Group.

Sinason, V. (2011b). Introduction. In V. Sinason (Ed.). *Attachment, Trauma and Multiplicity: Second Edition. Working with Dissociative Identity Disorder*, pp. 3–18. London: Routledge / Taylor and Francis Group, and Hove, East Sussex: Routledge / Taylor and Francis Group.

Sinason, V. (2011c). The Shoemaker and the Elves. In V. Sinason (Ed.). *Attachment, Trauma and Multiplicity: Second Edition. Working with Dissociative Identity Disorder*, pp. 127–138. London: Routledge / Taylor and Francis Group, and Hove, East Sussex: Routledge / Taylor and Francis Group.

Sinason, V. (2011d). Interview with Detective Chief Inspector Clive Driscoll. In V. Sinason (Ed.). *Attachment, Trauma and Multiplicity: Second Edition. Working with Dissociative Identity Disorder*, pp. 195–203. London: Routledge / Taylor and Francis Group, and Hove, East Sussex: Routledge / Taylor and Francis Group.

Sinason, V. (2012). Infanticide and Paedophilia as a Defence Against Incest: Work with a Man with a Severe Intellectual Disability. In J. Adlam, A. Aiyegbusi, P. Kleinot, A. Motz, and C. Scanlon (Eds.). *The Therapeutic Milieu Under Fire: Security and Insecurity in Forensic Mental Health*, pp. 175–185. London: Jessica Kingsley Publishers.

Sinason, V. (2020). *The Truth About Trauma and Dissociation: Everything You Didn't Want to Know and Were Afraid to Ask*. London: Confer Books.

Sinason, V. (2022a). Working with Primitive Bodily Communications in the Context of Unbearable Trauma in Non-Verbal Patients: Smell, Silence, and Winnie the Pooh. In R. Hilty (Ed.). *Primitive Bodily Communications in Psychotherapy: Embodied Expressions of a Disembodied Psyche*, pp. 51–61. London: Karnac / Karnac Books, Confer.

Sinason, V. (2022b). Chapter 2. In R. Hilty (Ed.). *Primitive Bodily Communications in Psychotherapy: Embodied Expressions of a Disembodied Psyche*, p. 207. London: Karnac / Karnac Books, Confer.

Sinason, V., and Conway, A. (Eds.). (2022). *Trauma and Memory: The Science and the Silenced*. London: Routledge / Taylor and Francis Group, and Abingdon, Oxfordshire: Routledge / Taylor and Francis Group.

Sinason, V., Hollins, S., Gillani, H., and Laird E. (2022). *A Refugee's Story*. London: Beyond Words / Books Beyond Words.

Wilson, S. (1998). *The Courage to Let Go: Disability and Psychotherapy*. M.A. in Psychotherapy and Counselling, City University, London, at the School of Psychotherapy and Counselling, Regent's College, Inner Circle, Regent's Park, London.

Chapter 3

How Working with Disabled People Can Make Us Better Psychotherapists

Shula Wilson

The human struggle with the inevitability of death leads people to embrace all that distracts them from their mortal nature and escape all that reminds them that they are eventually going to die. The damaged human body is one stimulus that often triggers death anxiety. This is probably the main reason why only very few psychotherapy training programmes and thus psychotherapists consider this seriously and devote time to understand the ways disability affects the psyche.

The disabled people who taught me the meaning of being an outsider

When I first came to England, I found the strangeness exciting and the unfamiliarity somehow felt comfortable. I happily exchanged the over familiar and at times suffocating atmosphere of my home country for the position of 'not belonging'.

I enjoyed the freedom of the anonymity. What I did not welcome about my experience in the new country was that everyone spoke English, which meant that I was unable to communicate. When I did summon enough courage to use the fragments of English I remembered from school, I found myself on a primitive plain; experiencing the frustration of a pre-verbal infant. My thoughts and ideas were of my adult self, I knew what I wanted to say but when I tried to put it into words it came out unintelligible.

I was not able to make myself understood. When, eventually I managed to muster enough English I found a job in a day centre for disabled people. Unbeknown to me at the time, this led me to become a psychotherapist specialised in disability. For a long time, I was puzzled by my choice. There is no link to disability in my background history; what is it that pulled me towards this client group? It took many years of analysis and self-processing to realise that attaching myself to a minority group as a non-member replicated my very early experience.

I was born in a budding Kibbutz, in Israel, which in those days, despite the hardship, was a close and warm community. Yet in strange contrast, the child-rearing regime prevented open expression of warmth and closeness; the

DOI: 10.4324/9781003646242-5

babies were separated from their parents, allowing only very limited and strictly controlled visiting and feeding time. A nursemaid, not the parents, was in charge. When I was about three, our Kibbutz disintegrated. My parents moved to a small town, and set up a family home into which my sister and brother were born. The little girl who was left to cry at night away from her parents was now watching how her siblings were being looked after by the very same parents, not by a nursemaid. Why was she not looked after by her parents? The only way she could find to quieten this disturbing question was to imagine herself as an alien, not really belonging.

This is probably why being actually a stranger felt so familiar – in a paradoxical way, I have arrived where I belong, and I belong with those who don't belong, who are aliens. This is also what I believe led me to become a professional outsider – a therapist interested to work with disabled people. It is not the impairment or disability that drew me towards this group; it is the alienation that is in common. I feel a strong sense of familiarity in the company of people who are condemned to exile within their own society and sometimes within their own family.

However, unlike people in exile who have a memory or even a legend of a homeland, people who have been born with impairment have no memory of a place to dream about or long for.

Lorna was one of the first disabled people I met in the day centre. She was a young woman in a wheelchair with a big bib to soak her dribble. The spasms and involuntary movements prevented her from controlling the use of her hands, which meant that she was dependent on others for feeding, toileting, washing, dressing and any other physical need she might have. Her speech was quite slurred, which made understanding and conversing with her difficult. I felt somewhat anxious, due to my perceived inability to communicate with Lorna. So, I reverted to the 'demand and control mode' and I started to ask questions. One of which was: '*If by magic you could be granted one thing, what would it be?*' I was expecting her to wish for the ability to walk or for the use of her hands, but what Lorna wished for was to have clear speech. This was a surprise, as I had not realised then, that impaired communication could be experienced by people with multiple disability as the worst aspect of their condition.

Elizabeth Greeley (1996), in her moving autobiography, writes:

> The part of my disability which causes me the most frustration is the way my speech and swallowing have been, and are, affected. This means that both communication through speech and socialising while having a meal are harder to carry out. In the past I have been very depressed about it.
>
> (Greeley, 1996, p. 97)

Not being able to communicate means isolation and frustration. Inflicting isolation and frustration on others are the widest used methods of punishment in the form of imprisonment and solitary confinement. Dostoyevsky's experience of penal servitude, according to Storr, permanently influenced his view of human nature. Seeing convicts, who for years had been ruthlessly crushed, suddenly break out and assert their own personalities, often in a violent and irrational fashion, made him realise that individual self-expression or self-realisation was a basic human need (Storr, 1997, p. 59). Dostoevsky observed people who were silenced by their environment: they possessed the physical ability to speak and express themselves, but their physical survival was dependent on suppression of self-expression. Yet, as Dostoevsky observed, there is a point when life loses its value without self-expression.

Di is paralysed apart for limited movement in her left hand. Due to lack of control of her facial muscles, Di cannot produce speech in the way most people use for communication. She can indicate without words 'yes' and 'no' and produce sounds that comes across as something between barks and baby talk. She knows the 'native language' English, yet, when trying to form relationship with her own folks she finds it very difficult because they can hardly decipher her communications.

Throughout the two years I worked with Di the themes that kept on weaving into the tapestry of our relationship were her loneliness and the longing to be loved.

Di is able to operate an electric wheelchair and a specially adapted computer with her left hand. In order for Di to operate the computer a wrist-switch has to be fastened to the palm of her left hand so she can press it with her fingers. For all other physical functions and needs she is entirely dependent on others.

Prior to my first session with Di, her occupational therapist (O.T.) approached me to say that she would set up Di's computer in the consulting room. She went on to explain that Di would not be able to communicate without the computer. The O.T.'s intervention had provoked my anxiety about Di before I had ever met her.

The first session was a trial for both of us. I was anxious about communicating with a client who could not produce clear speech. The presence of the computer disturbed me because I generally don't feel at ease with machines. It reminded me of those cubist paintings of Braque and Picasso, when the body is divided into its parts which are then spread all over the canvas. Di's mouth was on the table, in the form of the computer, separated from her body and linked by a wire to her wrist. Di was able to produce sounds when she was trying to speak, but they rarely sounded like words.

Everything that could go wrong went wrong. It was difficult to get the electric wheelchair into the room, then the wires came off and Di wanted me to call for the O.T. I listen to my instinct that told me to wait.

After a while I managed to gather my thoughts and was able to acknowledge the difficulties experienced by both of us, yet refraining from calling for help. Despite this shaky start Di was keen to embark on a therapeutic relationship with me, using the computer as an interpreter.

The first step towards building trust was resisting the temptation to call for help. The next was acknowledging my shortcomings and focusing on listening and decoding Di's messages.

One day, about five months into the therapy, I could not find the computer in its usual place. Di had indicated that it had been left on the ambulance. This felt like a challenge, not to have a third party. I have realised that I became accustomed to, and perhaps also dependent on the presence of the computer as a chaperon, keeping an eye on us. In the therapy room we kept the same arrangement, sitting side by side in front of the empty table, only this time we were looking at each other, rather than at the screen. I said: *'Perhaps the computer was left because you are a bit fed-up with it. Although the computer helps to be precise and accurate, it is also coming between us'.*

We struggled to communicate directly without the machine. I had to guess each word several times before I 'got it' and some words were probably lost or misunderstood. Di talked about her mother who died a year earlier and about her sister who had been busy, working too hard and Di was worried about her sister's health. We were able to communicate directly, without the computer. Di's comments may have also reflected her concern about the therapist working too hard.

Di has waited patiently for me to master the computer, only so that she could 'drop' it. It will be helpful at this point to examine this process from a developmental perspective. The computer had been invested with the role of a transitional object (Winnicott, 1960). Like a child who is using a doll to replace their mother until such time that dependency has turned into self-reliance, so was Di using the computer until she felt safe enough to trust herself in this new relationship. Only then was she able to let go of the inanimate object. Di kept on saying 'I feel lonely, I want to be happy'. I linked it to the communication difficulties, which I could not rectify; all that I could offer was to keep on struggling and staying with our mutual frustration.

Working with Di took me yet again, back to my first days in England when I did not believe anyone would understand me. I remember how cut off I felt when the phone rang and I would not pick it up for the fear that the person at the other end would be 'a native', one of those who could only speak English.

I, as a foreigner, and my clients as disabled people often are at the receiving end of the tendency to relate to people who are different and therefore seem not to belong, as if they are not fully grown adults. The image of the 'adult' as a whole object assumes an accomplished level of physical and mental functioning. When an individual is not performing to the level generally expected of adults, a question may arise as to whether or not this person is a 'real' adult, or more poignantly, is this 'being' really one of us? Is this a wrongly developed child, a monster, a cheat or pretence? Whichever way you look at it, the disturbance created by the presence of difference will remain, and may lead to defensive reaction, in the form of projecting primitive fear onto those perceived as different. This process of projective identification

(Klein, 1948), demonises differences, justifies persecution and activates pre-datory and existential death anxiety. Yet, perhaps living in-between two worlds has also a defensive 'cheating' quality. As a foreigner, I can change colours like a chameleon; if it suits me, I can pretend I don't understand, I can also use my 'foreignness' as a camouflage. Despite the rejection, there is still a choice and possibly some advantages. The most obvious one is developing and sharpening guessing skills.

The struggle to decode, understand and function within an environment that does not see you as a full member becomes a familiar part of everyday life, almost a second nature that creates the habit of regularly questioning one's understanding. It can also contribute towards a working awareness that what one hears is not always what has been said. The need to adapt to a new environment sharpens the ability to receive and respond to verbal and non-verbal cues and could enhance the way we decode unconscious messages.

Another benefit of being an outsider is 'a licence for ignorance' or the permission one is given by self or others for not knowing, which frees one from the pretence to know when you actually don't. This ignorant status paves the way toward a comparative ease at questioning and seeking clarification.

Through the story of Di, we can gain some understanding as to the way both client and therapist react to anxiety that is being evoked by the inability to interact through the use of language in direct vocal fashion to which the therapist is accustomed. The hypothesis is that the client's impaired speech heightens the therapist's anxiety because it leaves the therapeutic dyad exposed, bereft of the protective cover of language which, as well as being a means of communication and interaction, also offers defence options. It can hide thoughts and feelings as well as reveal them.

The next case study is the story of Michael.

Survival and its cost

On the phone was a woman asking if I could help her father. '*He is depressed*' she said, '*the GP prescribed anti-depressants which seems to have triggered frequent hallucinations and very morbid thoughts, says he wants to die. I am very worried about him*'.

Michael is 60 years of age, working part time in a public service as a skilled manual worker. He came to see me because of what he called 'panic attacks' which he described as severe trembling and uncontrollable shaking, weeping and unexplained haunting fears. The most disturbing symptom was the fear to stay inside his own home. Michael and his wife had moved to their new house about a year prior to commencing the counselling. The reasons for the move were to improve their living conditions and be near his two adult children and their respective families. But somehow it did not work, Michael felt that the neighbours were avoiding him, and he got himself involved in an unpleasant confrontation with a next-door neighbour about the drumming noise produced by a 15 year old boy. '*It is not like me*' he said. He could not bear staying in the house after sunset. He felt engulfed by hostility.

When I first met Michael, he was spending most of his free time at his daughter's home. He saw his inability to stay in his own house as his fault and a weakness, which fed into the anxiety caused by the fear that the house provoked.

Michael appears as a solid, polite and well-presented person who is able to articulate his thoughts in a clear and fluent manner.

He is the youngest of five children, the nearest siblings to him are twin brothers who were very close to each other, and little Michael was left alone and isolated.

They were all evacuated during the war. Soon after they came back, his mother left home to live with her own mother.

At this point I need to make a confession: the service that Michael was seeking counselling from is designated for people who are affected by disability, though Michael does not have any physical or other disability apart from his current neurosis. Strictly speaking, I should not have accepted him for counselling. How come I have found myself bending the rules for him? Yes, we were looking for more clients, but I still managed to turn away quite a few who did not meet the criteria. In reflection, I believe that his experience of isolation and loneliness echoed strongly with my outsiderness. He was a survivor who used to look after himself and others. I respected him for it. Once I realised boundaries had been broken it heightened my awareness to what appeared to be a subjective attitude, and I became vigilant in monitoring how this may affect our therapeutic relationship.

Michael was consumed by fear, and what made it unbearable for him was his inability to make any sense of it. He was terrified, but did not know what he was afraid of. A metaphor he used to describe his experience was: '*It is like when a computer goes all wrong, it just makes horrible noises and buzzes and fusses, and whatever knob you press, just makes it worse, it is being completely out of control, not being able to stop what is happening to you.*' At this early stage of therapy, I hardly intervened at all, I just stayed with him, listening, sometimes paraphrasing and reflecting. I felt as confused and unable to make sense of these experiences, as Michael did. His struggle to control his mind reminded me of Di's struggle to gain some control over her body.

Michael's early memories are of him and his brothers hiding under the table while his father beat his mother and threatened to kill her and the children. They lived in a poor but close community where everyone knew each other and care of children was shared. So when Michael managed to escape from his father, he invariably would find an open door nearby, to hide and if lucky to be offered some food and warmth. Then came the Second World War, Michael's father went away and both Michael and his siblings were evacuated to the country. The countryside was so different from anything he knew. He liked the open green spaces, the fresh air and the birds. But he was not sure how to be with the village children who did not welcome him. During the two years they stayed, his mother came only once; to tell them that their father had been killed in action.

About two months into the counselling Michael was talking about his feeling of dread and anger when hearing the news or reading a newspaper, because he was really worried about the young children who are being abused and sometimes disappear without trace. I could not see the link, I was puzzled. The next session, Michael started by talking about the war:

> *During the war, after we came back from the 'country' we had to live in the underground tunnels because of the 'blitz', my mother was a warden, she was making sure everything was right in our part of the tunnel. One evening I was out playing with some other kids, when a man came and ask me to show him where the telephone is, I did not think much of it and went along to show him. After a few steps he grabbed me into the bushes and was trying to do things to me. I did not understand what he was trying to do, but I knew it was not right. I was terrified but somehow, I managed to escape and run back to our part of the tunnel. My mother did not notice at all that I was missing, she was much too busy looking after other people, for her to pay any attention to me.*

He paused and then said: '*I could have been dead and nobody would have known. I never talked about it before, I never told anybody*'. For 52 years Michael was carrying alone the painful wounds caused by the fear, neglect and shame of the abuse. Telling his story was a first step towards a clue that was to lead to the cause of the fear that created the 'panic attacks'. According to Winnicott (1974, pp. 103–107), 'There is a big proportion of all people who successfully hide a need for a breakdown, the potential breakdown is awaiting an outside trigger'. The panic attacks could be seen as Winnicott's 'breakdown'. What was the trigger, and how does it link to the fear of being in his own home? The experience of the physical assault, at the age of eight was a traumatic event, as Laplanch and Pontalis (1973) define trauma. It was an experience that Michael could not absorb and therefore remained in his psyche as a 'foreign body'. The outcome of the trauma is always the incapacity of the psychical apparatus to illuminate the disturbing affect and to keep balance.

In an attempt to forget and start afresh, Michael suppressed his bad memories and never talked about his childhood. He was busy, finishing his education, finding work, looking after his young family, he was doing well and did not want to let the disturbing childhood memories interfere with his life. He was able, for a time, to encapsulate those thoughts and memories and push them to the very back of his mind. When his first beloved wife died, the capsule holding the past started to break and his memories were haunting him. After a few lonely years he married his second wife, hoping to keep the past at bay. But with the difficulties of a new relationship and ageing, the capsule burst and the raw unbearable childhood memories came back. He was thrown into an inner world where there is no safe place: violence and threats at home; rejection, abuse and neglect outside. In his mind his current home had become the home he needed to escape from as a child. Nothing was safe anymore; all was contaminated with fear and dread. The home became a symbol of deception, it was supposed to protect but instead there were threats and attacks.

Telling the 'secret', exposing the traumatising 'foreign-body' seemed to have been a turning point on several levels:

Michael and I survived it. He was not being punished for telling his tale and I was not 'shocked' into incapacity (although this carries its own disappointment as we will see later).

Also, by talking about the assault, the neglect and the emotions that he had experienced, Michael got in touch with the first 'clue' which led to some understanding and perhaps found some sense in, what felt at the time, a very chaotic space. Surviving the test of exposing his story and feeling understood, opened up the 'floodgate' and Michael was now able to talk freely about what came to his mind.

On a cold winter day Michael recalled:

> When we were in the county as evacuees, I went out with the others to play on the iced river, I can't remember how it all happened but suddenly I was under the ice in the freezing cold water, I felt trapped, I thought I will die there, I did not think anyone will come to get me out. They did, my sister saw me missing and shouted for help.

Here was yet another illustration of Michael experiencing fear, danger and feeling abandoned.

I shared with Michael my understanding, made a link between his childhood events that had been life threatening, and his current panic attacks. I suggested that it could be a delayed reaction, that when he actually experienced the frightening events he could not afford to acknowledge and react to the terror, because admitting weakness would have been too dangerous. Therefore, he had to 'freeze' his reaction and store it away. Only now, when he feels more or less secure and his children are not dependent on him anymore, has his unconscious 'allowed' the frozen reaction to thaw and to come up to the surface. Accepting this interpretation meant that Michael was feeling and reacting now to events that took place more than 50 years ago.

Being able to make sense seemed to reduce the symptoms. Michael was reporting an improvement in his everyday life; he could walk along the street without thinking that everyone was looking at him. He managed to stay in the house for the night and managed to stand up to his wife. The way he presented his wife echoed very much the way he experienced his mother. 'The return of the repressed.' I suggested the possibility that what attracted him to his wife could have been familiarity, as he observed in his wife many characteristics that were similar to his mother; a strong personality that often gives a double message, such as: ' *"This is my lovely baby"*, *to other people and then ignoring me*'. One of the complaints against his wife was that she did not understand him. It took me a long while to understand that he was also talking about me.

It was a session after the holiday and Michael arrived about five minutes late (he came late for several weeks prior to the holiday, which was very unlike him). He reported a panic attack when he was at home. His daughter and her family were there:

> *I was in a bad way, I went to the doctor and asked him to take me off the 'Prozac', it does not seem to help. I want something that will help me to cope...I had a fight with my wife, she is not helpful when I am not well, I did tell her I feel scared inside, but she just says, there is nothing to be scared of...I need to find a way to understand what it was, I was off my food, my stomach was in knots...*

Although he was talking about his wife, I could clearly hear his anger also directed at me. What had I done to trigger the images of people who are there to help and support, but actually they are not doing what they are supposed to do? I had disappointed him like I had disappointed Di, but how? And then 'the penny dropped'. Michael was trying to communicate to me through his lateness and I was not responding; I had ignored him. I was useless, like his mother, the wife and the doctor. When I finally acknowledged my failing to pay attention to his lateness as an expression of anger, Michael said: '*Maybe, I just want it all to go away, I want to be normal again, I need somebody who will understand me*'. I see this session as another breakthrough: Michael's anger was heard and acknowledged, and again, both of us survived it. The expression of anger did result neither in punishment nor in destruction. This session took part about a year into therapy, and there were no more panic attacks.

About three months later Michael moved house, leaving behind the house that made him so fearful and depressed. In his words he is '*happy, but not yet 100%*'. He is now revisiting his painful memories, but this time from a position of his newly acquired strength:

> *I remember running to the tube, I know it is real but I cannot remember anything after, if somebody would have only asked me where I was, but nobody did* [like me not noticing his lateness] ... *After I told you, then I told other people and I was surprised that nothing happened, they were not shocked.*

Michael is still not convinced that he is not going to be punished. But now he is able to own his life story, and he is beginning to seek his personal truth by separating phantasy from reality yet acknowledging they inter-relate. There are more dreams coming now about hitting and kicking his father or cutting his mother. Being able to remember the dreams seems to indicate regaining inner strength. Recently Michael reported that for the first time he asked to be paid for overtime. In the past he was afraid to ask for what was due to him. Now that he does not need to hide anymore, he is able to accept himself, and can confidently expect others to accept and respect him.

Michael is talking about *'The time when I would not have to come here anymore, when I will feel comfortable in my new house'*.

I believe that Michael's natural resilience and his ability for self-healing are the main contributors to his wellbeing. My part is mainly due to being aware of him as 'special' client, the special child he had never been. This led me to be particularly careful in maintaining and upholding the boundaries as best as I was able to.

Discussion: how can the experience of working with people with disability, such as Di inform and improve therapists' practice?

Let's start with communication: most therapists rely on verbal exchange as the main form of interaction with clients. The world of words is the therapist's comfort zone. Thus, working with people who have limited speech provides a challenging opportunity to develop the skills of listening to actions as if they were words. Di was not able to say she wanted us to look at each other, and that I should try to understand her speech. Her nonverbal way of communicating was to leave the computer behind. As for Michael, his unconscious was not ready to acknowledge and express how neglected he felt, so he acted out; he came late. The challenge was: 'Will the therapist notice my lateness/ absence? Or will my therapist ignore me like my mother did?'

I believe that the experience with people such as Di enabled me eventually to hear the message hidden in his lateness.

Di and other people who live with a damaged body helped me to see the parallel between the protective role of Body and that of Home, and to appreciate the painful struggle when one or the other is dysfunctioning. Gaining an insight into the experience of a damaged body provides a deeper understanding of the predicament of disadvantaged and vulnerable people such as the homeless, refugees and immigrants.

Confronting the reality of human helplessness

One of the reasons why most therapists shy away from working with disabled people is the dread of feeling helpless. Therefore, breaking through the fear barrier when experiencing close encounters with disabled people may help to confront helplessness and demystify the notion of disability, thus enhancing one's ability to deal with the challenges of human suffering in its full complexity of mind and body. The therapist's position as an outsider will enable withstanding this challenge. That means caring, but not getting involved, and holding onto an outside vantage point which provides a full view of the patient's life in its context. It also means keeping a distance that allows the therapist enough sense of safety so she can engage with the patient without feeling threatened by her inability to change the patient's predicament.

The French philosopher Maurice Merleau-Ponty (1962) suggested that the concept of the perfect body held in the mind is the 'wished for body', or the body as a whole, as opposed to the 'body at the moment' which is the body we actually possess, with all its imperfections. For disabled people the 'wished for body' is much further away than it is for non-disabled people. Yet, in my experience most disabled people accept the reality of their body. You may say, that is so because the temptation and opportunities to deny reality are fairly limited. Whatever the reason, there is a great deal we can learn from disabled people about accepting the given and challenging what can be challenged. Perhaps most important is facing personal truth and finding ways of making the most of one's life. Rather than complaining of what we don't have, living with disability is about accepting limitations and amongst them the reality of our limited body.

Working with disabled people provides ample opportunities to check our reactions, attitudes and self-awareness. Being somewhat surprised when Lorna wished for better speech, or when Di was longing for love made me aware of my own limited view and highlighted the fact (excuse the cliché) that regardless of the state of the body we all yearn for human contact and love.

When John, my client who is blind says: *'I do not want to be "the blind", I am a person who is also "blind"'*, he is illuminating and honouring pain or deformity as something separate from the person's identity.

Treating with respect, the motto of the Institute of Psychotherapy and Disability, is about a two-way relationship. The more obvious one is respecting the disabled client as a whole unique human being whose life is worth living. The others aspect is RE-spect: an invitation to therapists to take a second look to re-examine themselves, while keeping the outsider's vantage point.

Bibliography

Greeley, E. (1996). *The Unclear Path*. London: Hodder & Stoughton.
Klein, M. (1948). *Contribution to Psychoanalysis*. London: Hogarth Press.
Laplanch, J. and Pontalis, J-B. (1973). *The Language of Psychoanalysis*. London: Karnac.
Merleau-Ponty, M. (1962). *Phenomenology of Perception*. London: Routledge.
Storr, A. (1997). *Solitude*. London: HarperCollins.
Wilson, S. (2003). *Disability Counselling and Psychotherapy*. London: Palgrave Macmillan.
Winnicott, D. W. (1960). The theory of the parent-infant relationship. In: *The Maturational Process and the Facilitating Environment*. New York: International University Press.
Winnicott, D. W. (1974). Fear of breakdown. *The International Review of Psychoanalysis*, Volume 1, pp. 103–107. London: Routledge.

Working as a Disability Psychotherapist

Chapter 4

Du sei wie Du: About Love and Passion

Johan De Groef

My Choice

It wasn't my choice to work in the area of disability. I studied educational sciences, cultural anthropology and philosophy at the KU Leuven and training as a psychoanalyst in the Belgian School for Psychoanalysis followed. These studies were chosen and partly determined by my personal and family history. My initial interest was to work in a classical clinical setting and I also had a wish to write a PhD on the links between psychoanalysis and dialogal philosophy (Buber, Rosenzweig). Initially I had the intention to do my substitute military duty in Africa but on meeting the woman who became my wife I did it at the Institute for Fundamental Research of Law of KULeuven (Broekman 1996, 2016).

In the late 1970s there was a lot of unemployment so after my substitute military service I was searching for work. This was made even harder by my profile. A dream job seemed far away. *It was rather by accident, considered in retrospect a happy coincidence*, that I met Rudi Vermote (today a well-known psychoanalyst and Bion specialist) who was at that time medical director of OTB Kampenhout (a residential setting for adults with a learning disability). I could start as a pedagogue in his unit in the interim.

That was a revelation! 1986 was my *'gründerjahr'* in which I discovered the subject of disability.

At the same time that *'new' discovery* was for me also a *rediscovery*: a personal and theoretical revelation of something very familiar: on the one hand on my mother's side there were stories about some distant relatives and on my father's side there was an uncle with a learning disability. Additionally, theoretically, I held the psychoanalytic core idea (Freud's crystal principle: 1933, 15): nothing human is alien to me, however different that person may be.

From then, working in the field of disability was experienced by me as *feeling at home. The clinical encounter* with people with a learning disability and certainly those with so called 'behavioral problems' or/and mental health problems, became a close 'encounter of the first kind'. All that followed is history, as can be read in some of my writing (De Groef, 1999, 2011, 2021; De Groef and Vermote, 2015).

DOI: 10.4324/9781003646242-7

These experiences also inspired my work as a psychoanalyst in private practice for people without a learning disability. Thanks to my experiences with people with a disability, which is a truly psychoanalytic experience, the power of listening and talking became even more loud and clear.

So what at first seemed like a non-choice, a coincidence, revealed at second glance not only a happy coincidence, but *an unconscious choice*, a true encounter and a dream (job) that became reality. So it will not surprise you that the work makes me happy and that I am grateful to the people I've met.

Hallmarks of Disability Therapy

From a psychoanalytic point of view and in accordance with Freud's crystal principle (Freud, 1933) or Jacques Schotte's anthropopsychiatry (Schotte, 1990) – one of the founding fathers of the Belgian School for Psychoanalysis – psychotherapy with clients with a disability isn't essentially or structurally different from psychotherapy with any kind of patient. Of course there are differences, but in a quantitative and not in a qualitative way. As always, a therapist has to translate his/her framework in respect to the particular person with his/her problems and possibilities in front of him/her. Attunement in the therapeutic relationship and an attuned co-construction is necessary and indispensable.

Successful contact and a respectful reception of the person is essential and an acceptance of fragility knowing that a person with a disability has mostly a (long) history of exclusion. A psychoanalytic approach is a so-called inclusive approach because of that anthropopsychiatric principle expressed in the words of the Roman poet Terentius (163 BC): I am human, and I think nothing human is alien to me. That's the main reason why psychoanalytic therapy and certainly a psychoanalytically trained therapist fits well as a therapist for this client group. The personal analysis is a necessary condition to work through 'our dark continent' and all the themes which are often, without camouflage, projected into the therapeutic relation and framework and are brutally mirrored in our therapeutic face.

It is easy to make these points but in reality it requires a lot of work on our countertransference and our 'negative capability' (Keats, 1817) in order to understand and warmly receive a person who has survived the imbroglio of not being-desired, of being an unwelcome guest (Ferenczi, 1929; Van Coillie, 2004), a stranger.

A psychoanalytic approach and attitude is formulated by an 18th century romantic German folk-poem in the collection of *Des Knaben Wunderhorn* (Von Arnim and Brentano, 1806 /1923, 275):

> I give you something
> What would you like?
> A silver wait-a-while
> And a goulden nothing
> In a never-before-seen box.

A Flemish proverb states: 'unknown is unloved'. The best way to begin an acquaintance is – as I experienced myself – to have the 'ethical' and professional obligation to start and to experience the challenge and the wealth that is returned. Therapists must overcome their fear of the unknown to survive the narcissistic injury of feeling helpless.

Listening to people who speak with few words, 'listening to whispering', requires not only a scientific training but also a background of reading literature and especially poetry, which creates a whole world with few words. The therapeutic cleared-out imagination is essential for life and also the therapeutic life. Psychoanalytic therapy with a person with a learning disability should be an integral part of the general psychoanalytic and psychotherapeutic training.

What are the human themes which appear so magnified on the therapeutic stage?

The disability itself
The de-idealisation and the experience of loss
The experience of being in the throes of dependency
Sexuality and the procreative desire for 'successors'
The fear of being excluded or even killed

So it is overwhelmingly clear that these are not subjects to which simple answers are possible. On the contrary, these are themes to articulate to the slow rhythm of the person with a learning disability and to work through in a safe, coherent therapeutic relationship. A safe containing contact remains the basic requirement in addition to the being there – even with a lot of silences and few words from the therapist. A face to face sitting setting is not easy. Unsurprisingly, therapeutic walking can help with this. Not face to face but side by side moving forwards. Wondering and wandering help as if both are searching members of the Aristotelian philosophical peripatetic school.

To conclude this section with a poem (my own translation) of the Flemish poet Leonard Nolens (2004, p. 597):

Let
Slow
Slow.
Slow your step.
Step slower than your heartbeat demands.
Ease
Ease.
Ease your desire.
And disappear in moderation.
Do not take your time
And let time carry you away –
Let.

Passion and Love

I wish to preface this section with some philosophical thoughts on love.

'Whereof one cannot speak, thereof one must be silent', is Wittgenstein's (1922) last sentence in his *Tractatus Logico-Philosophicus*. But Love is a verb; with the emphasis as well on the act of doing something, i.e. on the 'work' as on the 'word' itself; love is above all a word that works. No coincidence then that most jokes and songs are about love and love's pangs.

Yet it is poetry that through its shortage of words is flexible enough to talk about love in a concealing-revealing way. Poets are eternal lovers. They are in love with their beloved and with the language, but most of all perhaps with love itself that keeps inspiring them without end.

Paul Celan – a Romanian-Jewish German-speaking poet – wrote a poem (in the collection of poems *Lichtzwang*, 1970) with the opening words: *Du sei wie Du*: be yourself, or translated litterally – less beautiful but more correct – you be like you (Felstiner, 1983).

> DU SEI WIE DU, immer.
> (YOU BE LIKE YOU, always.)
> Auch wer das Band zerschnitt zu dir hin,
> (The very one who slashed the bond unto you)
> Knüpfte es neu, in der Gehugnis,
> (knotted it new, in myndignesse)
> Schlammbrocken schluckt ich, im Turm,
> (Spills of mire I swallowed, inside the tower)
> Sprache, Finster – Lisene.
> (Speech, dark-selvedge)

What is the meaning of 'be yourself' – what does: be as a you, as another, mean? Does Celan want to make clear that 'be yourself' means: be as – or resemble another ('yourself' seems indeed to resonate with self – the same – the identical) or does he mean 'to be yourself' is: to be different?

The casualness with which our culture appeals to us to be ourselves seems to be problematic in more than one way. By experience we know that being yourself is rather a task than a fact – it is not our given nature.

A perpetual theme when love is concerned is: how different may partners be, how similar must partners be so that a love affair can be called a real relationship? It certainly is not a coincidence that both in popular speech and in theory there exist two models – two views: a couple should consist of two of the same kind (we look among our own kind) or the other way round: a couple should consist of two opposites attracting one another. This looks like the chemistry of partner-choice; significantly Goethe (1809) speaks about W*ahlverwandschaften*.

In the next pages I should like to study in depth this theme out of my experiences with adults with intellectual disability.

Maybe you will be frowning and you will not be able to identify well enough with our client group to accept that they too would and could hold up to you a mirror of recognition.

Intellectually disabled people are genii in the art of adapting themselves and conforming to what others ask and expect of them. With Sinason I could call it a mask with an idiotic smile (Sinason, 1986). Very often they form – more than anyone else – a mirror, a screen for the things that keep us busy: ideas, expectations, illusions, not yet assimilated experiences etc.: but we do not listen to them.

In every reflection, we present ourselves – mostly unconscious of the fact that we do so – in such a way that others (people with intellectual disability) must follow our example. The one in front of us, then, is our mirror. We shut it out however and forget that the other is a reflection – we think that we are not looking into a mirror, but through a window; we have the feeling that we see an image and not a reflection. The surprise and the fear therefore are great when we realise the other happens to be a real other person. In metaphorical language: when we discover that the window is a mirror and experience how the other smashes our mirror to pieces, we suddenly look into the other's face (Levinas 1974, p. 159).

These mirror-experiences form the basis for integration or segregation – for Eros and Thanatos. The mirror on the wall is a key part in the fairy tale of every human being. The answer we give is the basis for peace or war.

Freud (1933, p. 15) spoke about the crystal principle, indicating by it that in pathology we get an extreme – monstrous – drawing of the thing which in so-called normal life appears in a balanced, but disguised form. Nothing human is unfamiliar to us; let us therefore try to take these words seriously and look the stranger, that the human being with an intellectual disability is, in the face and listen to what he tells us about ourselves in a whispering voice, even sometimes without words.

About Conception and Concepts

'Sexuality from the cradle to the grave' was the title of a previous congress on this theme. With the following case/experience I move upstream to the well (Magris, 1988) or more precisely to the images we have of the well(s).

Case I

Natascha is a 24 year-old woman with a severe intellectual disability. She hardly speaks – utters a few yells only. She is very lively, almost agitated and displays a lot of so-called behavioural problems at home: aggression against her mother, pulling out her hair etc. The aetiology of the disability is unknown.

She is the youngest of four children. Her mother is 56 years old (she was 32 when she became pregnant with Natascha) and she has always been a housewife; her father – of Russian origin – is 58 years old and has been working as an employee at an insurance company until recently.

During a discussion he tells us about the heavy inconvenience of having a disabled child: 'it is like having a traffic accident whilst being within the law; if I had arrived 10 minutes earlier or later at the junction, I would not have been involved in the accident'.

This man expresses what can be overheard between the lines in so many talks – what unconsciously lives in the mind of so many parents. Some thoughts come to mind as a result of this.

Why do parents want children?

Children are the continuation of their parents. Personal mortality – finiteness of life and the fundamental human shortcoming that nobody is perfect, is difficult to accept. We try to neutralize that in different ways. Children are thereby the preferential 'removers' – the bearers of the shortcoming, of that mortality. Like works of art, they are signed. They get the name of their creators and lead – just like works of art – after and next to the creators an independent life.

Children and time: the memory – the recollection as a substitute for love.

The being that we expect is not real; ' There is no such thing as a baby' (Winnicott 1987, p. 99). Natascha's parents had, as all parents have, so many beautiful and hopeful expectations. The brute reality (Lacan's concept of the 'Real/Reel', Lacan [1964/1973]), the birth of a child with a learning disability cannot be expressed in words. The obvious defect – shortcoming – extra 'handicap' upon the fundamental human shortcoming, breaks the mirror of the beautiful play (Sausse, 1996; Korff Sausse and Scelles, 2017). The piece of art has been damaged, one could say.

Such an experience could be called, after Freud (1919), an unheimlich (uncanny) experience: the most trusted person (a child as the continuation of yourself, your own flesh and blood) who at the same time is the most alien being. The metaphor of the traffic accident indicates the difficulty in feeling responsible for something you are only partly responsible for, something you are not to be blamed for. And yet there is the smouldering question of who is guilty?

No guilt or genetic fault?

Do I control my genes, what are the rules of biological intercourse and am I accountable?

Lacan (1960/1991) describes 'loving' as *'donner ce qu'on n'a pas'*. One of the meanings of this cryptic saying is that we – having a body and being a body – are not 100% self-responsible and master of our relationships let alone love relationship. We are not perfect/complete. The foundation of our existence comes from the other one – we are being carried. Nature is the hole in our culture. Our genes are not our genes in the same way that our children are not our children (Gibran, 2014). Responsibility is to take care for what is not our belonging.

It is a lifelong task to accept this responsibility as my responsibility in spite of all aggression and lack of power. It's an act of adoption and hospitality towards another, a '*Du*'.

The others are to blame not I. In this way the unbearable is made liveable; even if the culprit is only a fictitious offender: the genes, the doctor, the partner, the child itself etc. The child being the wrongdoer is of course the most unbelievable and most repressed possibility. Childish innocence itself getting the blame.

Nevertheless this big disillusionment – broken illusion – is dealt with in various ways. There are two dominant patterns returning in many variations: fathers more than ever immersing themselves into their work (waiting in the car park) and mothers escaping into overconcerned care (the passionate-aggressive care). A manic and a depressive form of dealing with loss. Both patterns are variations of Octave Mannoni's (Mannoni 1982, p. 113) '*le passioné: ne veut rien savoir*; I know, but…'.

Situation 2

Natascha causes problems mainly at home. The relationship with her mother escalates towards aggression within a few days. Natascha claims her mother makes her run for everything and nothing. She terrorizes everyone – especially her mother – with all kinds of caprices. When her mother does not react immediately Natascha gets angry and pulls her mother's hair. When they bring her back to the home and she has to leave her mother Natascha holds her mother tight as if she had become one with her. There is no other way but action.

Contractions and being reborn again and again, it looks as if Natascha is caught between a homesickness for completeness/fusion and longing for a place of her own (in the Institute she cheers up). A place of her own: what else can it mean but a place where her individuality – her being different – is accepted without any shadow (of the past)?

But to create that place, mother has to be good enough. For Winnicott (1987) 'good enough' means: not complete (not full, not empty). This means: less full and thus less empty (there is a pun in the Flemish '*vol*(full)-*ledig* (empty) while '*volledig*' means complete).

In the Antwerp Middelheimpark there is a statue by Pablo Gargallo: the prophet. It is an iron construction full of holes, but thanks to these holes and the vision gained through them a full expression of a moved and moving human being is created. Too much of a thing destroys its possibilities. The power of poetry says as much as possible with a few words. In the same way that there exists a negative architecture, there could be a negative pedagogy: a pedagogy that creates emptiness – a vacuum in which and by which a person can rise. Remember the potter who makes a pot: he turns/creates a paper-thin boundary that encloses emptiness.

This allows us to see the crucial role of the relation between man and woman, between father and mother and the children. The relation between father and mother is important for either an uplifting or a suffocating parent-child relation. When the relationship between man and woman wastes away and the father, for example, accepts that the mother is only interested in her child, then mother and child are drawn into a scorching *fata morgana*.

Case 2

Fabienne is a severely intellectually disabled woman of 29 years who has been living in the home for nine years. She is the oldest of 3 children. The aetiology of the intellectual disability is unknown. The *DSM-V* speaks about a diffuse developmental disturbance. Already in the kindergarten class a retarded psycho-motor development could be recognised; there was however a normal speech development.

Fabienne caused problems of aggression especially towards female companions, more precisely towards one of them: Griet. When Griet retired the same problems then occurred with the companion Fabienne met first.

Fabienne was so attached to Griet she could not bear to live without her and therefore she always looked for her company; separation was for Fabienne a place of horror. In her approach to Griet she became more and more demanding and this turned into aggression immediately. As a consequence Griet ran away and so the traumatic circle was reactivated.

In his play *A Midsummer Night's Dream* Shakespeare (1596/1976) writes how Oberon dribbles the juice of a flower on Titania's eyes, in order to make her fall in love with the first man she will see.

Love will scorch your heart...

This is a literary account of Freud's thematic development of the idea that the relation between mother and child (mother being the first woman you see when you open your eyes) is the prototype of all coming love affairs. In one of the Wednesday Seminars (Nunberg and Federn, 1981, p. 50) Freud says: '*Das Geheimnis der Liebe gipfelt in der Forderung, so geliebt zu werden, wie man als Kind von der Mutter geliebt worden ist*' (The secret of love lies in the demand to be loved in the same way you were once loved by your mother).

Fabienne was so in love with Griet that she would consume/eat her. This means to get physical possession of someone, because you are possessed by somebody. You have to go where the bread is buttered. A passionate affair is a relationship that does not tolerate any interspace; everything happens in the immediate proximity and is instantaneous. Love – also passionate love – is a struggle with space and time. The other one is expected to be perfect, to be present at any moment and all places. The other one is my God whom I worship. In a passionate love affair the past, the present and the future are pulled together into a universal moment: Freud speaks about a 'normal psychosis' (Freud 1916–1917, college XXVI). Such omnipotence and omnipresence lead to destruction and self-destruction. Coincidence is impossible and the passionate lover gets entangled in his own meshes.

'In the eyes of all lovers the idea of pure and blind coincidence seems blasphemy. Things that were not in the stars are meaningless' (De Wispelaere 2002, p. 43). That's why anxiety, fear and aggression, as a consequence of the loss of and the chasing away from 'the garden of Eden', also have a self-neutralizing effect. They destroy the nets and sets the prisoner free.

It is not surprising therefore that true love can only flourish in this paradox: to really love someone is letting him go. A real actualization of this paradox, implicates the setting up of a language. (Many behavioural problems of people with intellectual disability cease to exist, when we start speaking and listening – not discussing.)

Case 3

Eddy is a 34-year-old man with a moderate learning disability. He speaks rather well, but has only a limited vocabulary. Here too the aetiology of the disability is unknown.

At a certain moment Eddy is physically and mentally very busy about 'his girl' Anita. It is remarkable that he does not try to contact her, but boasts about her and his affair with her.

The actual presence of the other person (Anita) and their being together don't seem relevant here. It is an image of Anita that is present. Moreover, saying that 'Anita is his girl' is a speech act.

In linguistic philosophy this means that saying 'I love you' is not the description of a preceding reality, namely the act of loving you, but in saying the words 'I love you' that reality is created, the real thing is materialized.

Case 4

Sonja is a 28-year-old woman with a moderate learning disability. She has Down's syndrome. For about 6 years she had an affair with Guido, a man of 28 who also had a moderating intellectual disability – the aetiology of his disability was not known. Every day they both came from their own houses to the daycare centre. In the afternoon they used to sit hand in hand in their own psychological space in a hall with many people passing by.

One day Guido was killed in an accident. To the moral horror of the attendants and others the next day Sonja was found sitting hand in hand with another man with an intellectual disability. Is it that true love is not a thing of the moment?

Maybe Sonja was so full of Guido that the loss of him was unbearable for her at that moment. The vacuum had to be filled up. The person with an intellectual disability with his intellectual deficiency and therefore also the deficiency of memory has more difficulties in mourning through remembrance. Think of Freud's words in *Mourning and Melancholia* (Freud, 1917), or Joseph Brodsky in his own manner: if there is any substitute for love, it is memory. "To store something in your mind is therefore the restoration of an intimacy" (De Wispelaere 2002, 71). Sonja cannot get over and forget the loss of her friend, because she cannot remember him; or, writing verses in person:

> Nameless feelings
> Gnaw my skin
> Away
> Waving longing
> To see you yet
> > (J. De Groef)

Another person took the place of the remembrance – a man who resembled Guido in a certain way. Real love – certainly a very loyal love, may be unbearable holding love.

Case 5

Annouck is a woman of 28 with a mild to moderate intellectual disability. She is the eldest of three children. In the home where she stayed she was described as a nymphomaniac, who was addicted to affairs: at a party she used to fall in love with several men at the same time. At home Annouck is excluded and has almost no contact with her family. She is the stranger – the ugly duckling – in their midst.

This case seemed to be completely different from the previous ones. There are indeed several differences, but: does Annouck not enact the difficulty to cope with and accept her self? Is she not trying to forget the original loss – for her as a learning-disabled woman an even more dramatic loss – by starting new 'love affairs'?

In order to be able to love someone and be able therefore to let him go without fear of losing him, you must be held in the first place – someone must love you first. Leaving home is possible only when you have got a home, otherwise you drift away in the literal and figurative sense. Perhaps it is this passionate urge we can trace back to Annouck and so many other people with an intellectual disability. They are not these laughing and spontaneous people we believe them to be. Behind these smiling 'personas' there is a different world: a passionate drifter waiting for true words. The learning disabled man has left his motherland and is waiting in no man's land to be admitted in the promised land.

Lacan's (1960/1991) *'donner ce qu'on n'a pas'* (give what one does not have) also means: give space – space not yet filled up. In a Japanese way (think of the Japanese gardener who rearranges the stones and the sand of his garden every morning): build on sand and in that way keep alive the anticipation of the unexpected – no matter how small or strange it may be. The gesture of a potter who creates space: the hospitality of a pot.

Love in a Time of Loneliness (Verhaeghe, 1999). In this title the author makes a contraction of *One Hundred Years of Solitude* (Márquez, 1998) and *Love in the Time of Cholera* (Márquez, 1988). The words 'a hundred years' and 'cholera' have been left out. And so starts the story of Oedipus. Maybe like him we are condemned to answer the riddle of the Sphinx again and again: what is a human being? The final question for the panel to the Leitmotiv joins in with the Greek myth of Theseus. The thread of Ariadne led Theseus out of the labyrinth. The labyrinth thereby might be a symbol of the confusion of tongues after Adam and Eve, who had eaten the fruit of the tree of knowledge of good and evil, were chased out of the Garden of Eden. Since then, as Hölderlin writes in his poem 'Mnemosyne' (Beissner and Schmidt, 1969, p. 199):

Ein Zeichen sind wir,deutungslos,
Schmerzlos sind wir und haben fast
Die Sprache in der Fremde verloren.
(A token we are, without meaning,
Insensitive to pain we are and have almost
Lost the language/our tongue in foreign parts)
(my translation)

In this confusion we remain condemned to speak and are thrown together. This is the dimension of ethics and not of morals, or as in Hölderlin's 'Friedensfeier' (Beissner and Schmidt, 1969, p. 166):

Seit ein Gespräch wir sind
Und hören können voneinander.
(Since we are a talk we belong to
And can hear each other.)
(my translation)

Bibliography

Beissner, F. & Schmidt, J. (Eds.) (1969). *Hölderlin Werke und Briefe. Erster Band Gedichte Hyperion.* Frankfurt/Main: Insel Verlag.

Broekman, J. (1996). *Intertwinements of Law and Medicine.* Centre for Advanced Legal Studies Leuven, K.U., Leuven: Leuven University Press.

Broekman, J. (2016). *Meaning, Narrativity and the Real. The Semiotics of Law in Legal Education* IV. Frankfurt/Main: Springerverlag.

De Groef, J. & Heinemann, E. (Eds.) (1999). *Psychoanalysis and Mental Handicap.* London: Free Association Books.

De Groef, J. (2011). Psychoanalyse en Handicap, in J. Dirkx et al. (Ed.), *Handboek Psychodynamiek. Een verdiepende kijk op psychiatrie en psychotherapie.* Utrecht: De Tijdstroom.

De Groef, J. & Vermote, R. (Eds.) (2015). *Verstandelijke beperking en Psychoanalyse. Echo's van verlangen.* Antwerpen-Apeldoorn: Garant.

De Groef, J. (2021). 'Al wat geen helen kan verdragen, moet men strelen'. Enkele psychoanalytische reflecties bij 'langdurige zorg'. *Tijdschrift voor Psychoanalyse & haar toepassingen,* jrg.27, nr 2. Amsterdam: Boom Tijdschriften.

De Wispelaere, P. (2002). *Het verkoolde alfabet.* Amsterdam: Uitgeverij Atlas.

Felstiner, J. (1983). Paul Celan in Translation "Du sei wie Du". *Studies in 20th Century Literature,* 8(1) Special Issue on Paul Celan. Bloomington, IN:Indiana University Press.

Ferenczi, S. (1929/1984). *Das unwillkommene Kind und sein Todestrieb, in Bausteine zur Psychoanalyse, Band III: Arbeiten aus den Jahren 1908–1933.* Frankfurt/Main: Ullstein Materialien Ullstein Buch Nr 35205.

Freud, S. (1916–1917). A general introduction to Psycho-Analysis, *The Standard Edition of the Complete Psychological Works of Sigmund Freud,* Volume XV-XVI. London: The Hogarth Press.

Freud, S. (1917). Mourning and Melancholia. *The Standard Edition of the Complete Psychological Works of Sigmund Freud,*Volume XIV. pp.237–258. London: The Hogarth Press.

Freud, S. (1919). *The Uncanny,* Collected Papers IV. London: The Hogarth Press.

Freud, S. (1933). New introductory lectures on Psycho-Analysis. *The Standard Edition of the Complete Psychological Works of Sigmund Freud,* Volume XXII, pp.1–182. London: The Hogarth Press.

Gibran, K. (2014). *De Profeet.* Utrecht: Kosmos Uitgevers.

Goethe, J. W. (1809/1977). Die Wahlverwandschaften. Ein Roman. *Sämtliche Werke, Band* 9. München: Artemis Verlag, Deutscher Taschenbuch Verlag.

Keats, J. (1817/1931). Letter to George and Thomas Keats, in M. B. Forman (Ed.), *The Letters of John Keats.* London: Oxford University Press.

Korff Sausse, S. & Scelles, R. (Eds) (2017). *The Clinic of Disability: Psychoanalytical Approaches.* London: Karnac.

Lacan, J. (1964/1973). *Le Séminaire livre XI. Les quatre concepts fondamentaux de la psychanalyse.* Paris: Ed. du Seuil.

Lacan, J. (1960/1991). *Le Séminaire livreVIII. Le Transfert.* Paris: Ed. du Seuil.

Levinas, E. (1974). *Totalité et Infini. Essai sur l'exteriorité.* La Haye: Martinus Nijhoff.

Magris, C. (1988). *Donau. Een ontdekkingsreis door de beschaving van Midden-Europa en de crisis van onze tijd.* Amsterdam: Uitgeverij Bert Bakker.

Mannoni, O. (1982). *Ça n'empêche pas d'exister.* Paris: Ed. du Seuil.

Márquez, G. G. (1988). *Love in the Time of Cholera.* New York: Alfred Knopf.

Márquez, G. G. (1998). *One Hundred Years of Solitude.* Norwalk: Easton Press.

Nolens, L. (2004). *Verzamelde Gedichten. Laat alle deuren op een kier.* Amsterdam: Em. Querido's Uitgeverij.

Nunberg, H., & Federn, E. (Eds). (1981). *Protokolle der Wiener Psychoanalytischen Vereinigung. Band IV 1912–1918.* Frankfurt/Main: Fischer Verlag.

Sausse, S. (1996). *Le Miroir Brisé. L'enfant handicapé, sa famille et le psychanalyste.* Paris: Calmann-Lévy.

Schotte, J. (1990). *Szondi avec Freud. Sur la voie d'une psychiatrie pulsionnelle.* Bibliothèque de Pathoanalyse, Bruxelles: De Boeck-Wesmael.

Shakespeare, W. (1596/1976). *A Midsummer Night's Dream. Complete Works.* London: Oxford University Press.

Sinason, V. (1986). Secondary mental handicap and its relationship to trauma . *Psychoanalytic Psychotherapy 2(2)*, 131–154.

Van Coillie, F. (2004). *De Ongenode Gast. Zes psychoanalytische essays over het verlangen en de dood.* Amsterdam: Uitgeverij Boom.

Verhaeghe, P. (1999). *Love in a Time of Loneliness.* Montreal: Rebus Press.

Von Arnim, A. & Brentano, C. (Eds.) (1806/1923). *Des Kaben Wunderhorn. Alte deutsche Lieder gesammelt von Achim von Arnim und Clemens Brentano.* Frankfurt/Main: Suhrkamp, Insel Taschebuch 85.

Winnicott, D. (1987). *Through Paediatrics to Psycho-Analysis.* London: The Hogarth Press.

Wittgenstein, L. (1922). *Tractatus Logico-Philosophicus.* London: Routledge & Kegan Paul.

Chapter 5

Seeking Custody, Post Custody
Applying Disability Psychotherapy Thinking in the Criminal Justice System

Richard Curen

Introduction

Over the last 30 years disability psychotherapy, as described by Valerie Sinason (1992), Anne Alvarez (1992), Alan Corbett (2014) and colleagues (Corbett, Cottis and Morris 1996), Pat Frankish (2016), and others, has emerged as a discipline that provides us with critical tools and profound new ways of understanding the intellectually disabled, those with autism and those with physical disabilities. The development of this new field has much to offer non-disability, neurotypical focused fields and it is hoped that within this chapter there will be ideas that can illuminate those who write court reports in support of both victims and perpetrators of violence. As is found in the field of forensic psychotherapy, as described by Rosenfeld (1971), Welldon (1992, 2011), Glasser (1996) and Kahr (2002, 2020), the victim *and* the perpetrator are one and the same and exist in all of us to a greater or lesser degree. Thereby in both fields arbitrary delineations between disabled and non-disabled, and between victim and perpetrator, deny the oneness of these positions. It is well described in the disability psychotherapy field that non-disabled and neurotypical people project the disabled parts of themselves into others in order to make themselves feel more whole. Crucially though, it is most helpful to remember that the world can be divided into two distinct groups; the *disabled* and the *temporarily-able*, as almost all of us will become disabled at some point before we die.

I was blessed to work alongside Alan Corbett at Respond from 2002 and then later as one of his supervisees. Alan was the most wonderful mentor and guide in the complex and often strange intersections of the worlds of psychotherapy and of intellectual disabilities. I work as a 'forensic disability psychotherapist' which is a term Alan coined in his ground-breaking writing, particularly in his book *Disabling Perversions* (Corbett 2014). Alan was a guiding light in terms of thinking, assessment, treatment, supervision and training in the field of forensic disability psychotherapy and his untimely death was a personal loss but more importantly a loss to the world in terms of his thinking and its impact on patients and practitioners.

DOI: 10.4324/9781003646242-8

For me disability psychotherapy means treating patients with deep, genuine respect and recognising the often-devastating impact of deprivation and trauma, particularly the impact on attachment. It is also about finding new and innovative ways in which to engage patients who are initially hostile or suspicious of psychotherapeutic approaches, particularly psychodynamic ones.

Disability Psychotherapy Applied to Work in the Criminal Justice System

The criminal justice and mental health systems often fail to understand how forensic patients are almost always victims of violence well before they ever hurt themselves or anyone else. Clinicians working in these areas are often called upon to assess and make sense of actions and enactments that appear to have either a simple root cause, for example, when an offence is the re-enactment of an experience, they themselves have already suffered; or when the enactment appears to have no cause at all, for example, when the offence has no discernible aetiology. My belief is that the application of disability psychotherapy thinking can add insights to those clinicians whose practice includes working in the criminal justice system. This can be achieved by adding a foundation that builds on the central tenets of disability psy-chotherapy: respect, the ubiquitous presence of trauma, acute awareness of cultural differences, the importance of maintaining and paying attention to ruptures at the boundaries, paying attention to the unconscious (especially transference and countertransference) communications, and finally being creative in our approaches to our work. Building on Corbett's thinking I wish to discuss some clinical assessment material that throws up some of the challenges facing clinicians who are commissioned to write reports for court.

Clinical Illustration[1]

Bryony was referred to a community forensic service at the age of 36. She was going through the court process of trying to regain parental rights over her nine-month-old baby and hoped to later regain custody of her other two children, aged 16 and 14, who had both been placed in foster care. Six years previously, Bryony had been arrested and convicted of two sexual offences against the son of her neighbour. The neighbour had contacted the police when their 12-year-old son alleged that Bryony had sexually assaulted him.

Background

Bryony was the eldest of three children and had grown up with her parents in a home that was full of neglect, with a violent and alcoholic father and a depressed mother. Bryony did not get on with her father and had complicated relationships with her younger brother and sister. A combination of factors meant that Bryony struggled at school and she left with no qualifications. When she was 16 years old, she met a man called Alex with whom she had two children, a boy and then a girl. Alex was sadistic and cruel towards Bryony. He would force her to walk around the house naked, to engage in sexual activity with his male friends and at once coerced Bryony and her mother to engage in sexual activity together. Years of intimidation, using violence and the threat of further violence, led to Bryony becoming a sexual and domestic slave for Alex, to do with what he wanted. Alex would often photograph, or video Bryony and threatened to upload the material to force her to do more humiliating and degrading acts.

Index Offence

When Bryony and Alex's children were 10 and 8 years old, they would often play with their male neighbour who was 12 years old. One day when the neighbour was visiting and their own children were out of the room Alex encouraged Bryony to sexually touch the boy, which she did. Alex also encouraged the boy to touch Bryony which he did. Later the boy told his mother about what had taken place and she called the police and both Bryony and Alex were arrested. Their two children were immediately placed in foster care. Alex and Bryony went to court and both parents were sentenced to two years in prison. Bryony blamed Alex for coercing and intimidating her into committing the sexual offences against the neighbour. The judge found them both to be equally responsible.

Release

Neither parent had contact with each other but upon release from prison they both had supervised access to their children on different days, on a weekly basis. Bryony was placed on the Sex Offenders Register and was subject to a Sexual Harm Prevention Order (SHPO) that restricted her contact with children and meant that she was banned from residing with any person under the age of 18.

The New Couple

Bryony soon started a relationship with a man called Leo, who had no children of his own and who was a recovering drug addict. He had a long police record for drug-related offences and had two convictions for violence against adult men. Leo also came from a chaotic home. He was placed in children's homes from a young age, and it was there that he was sexually abused. Leo spoke about how he hated paedophiles and would not think twice before hurting one. Leo's hatred did not overtly apply to Bryony, herself a convicted paedophile.

Bryony soon fell pregnant, but the child was still born. There was lots of concern from social care professionals when she was pregnant, as the Sexual Harm Prevention Order (SHPO) prohibited her from living with any children. The still birth was a deeply upsetting experience for Bryony and Leo, while some professionals involved in the case described a sense of relief. They decided not to try again for another child but after about four years of being together Bryony became pregnant a second time.

The New Baby

Towards the end of the pregnancy Bryony became ill with anxiety and stress as she feared the child would either be still born again, or if it lived it would be removed from their home and placed in the care of the local authority. Leo was adamant that no child of his would go through the same experiences he had had as a child in care and therefore set about instructing solicitors to challenge the SHPO so that they might be able to parent their child themselves. The child was born healthy and was immediately placed with a foster carer. Bryony and Leo had three contact visits each week and both started to develop strong bonds with the baby, even though she was not able to live with them.

The Court Instructions

Bryony's solicitor contacted the forensic service in order to commission a court report that it was hoped would assess the level of risk Bryony might pose to her baby and to her other two children, if she were given parental responsibility again. Bryony was going through the court process to be able to have her baby living with her. The local authority's social workers were particularly concerned about the risk Bryony might pose to her baby if her baby were to return to her and Leo's care. Before the court report started, the lawyers for the local authority, for the baby and for each of the parents agreed that the assessment should take place over six weeks and should be funded from public funds.

The lawyers for the local authority were most alert to the impact of Bryony's previous sexual offences. There was a collective sense that although Bryony had sexually offended against a child, social services had let the family down and there was hope that this assessment would provide the court with a strategy and way forward. There was a sense of 'magical' thinking that by bringing in 'the experts' things would become much easier and the high levels of anxiety that were present would fade away. It was essential for the assessors working on the case to provide a level of containment needed in order to undertake the work, but to also be careful not to allow a fantasy to emerge that would allow a false sense of security.

Assessment Sessions

Weekly sessions with Bryony and Leo were organised and took place over six weeks, firstly in their home and then in the clinic. A meeting with Bryony's mother was also organised and took place at her home. The court papers and other documents that were made available painted a picture of a family that had experienced multiple traumas with competing and conflicting needs at every level and from all members of the family. The written material made it clear there was a long history of family neglect, trauma and abuse, the details of which were hard to digest, and it was easy to 'forget' the deeply affecting details of enacted aggression, sexual perversion and violence described over many years.

During the assessment sessions my colleague and I spoke at length individually with Bryony and then together with Leo about Bryony's offending history. Bryony presented in an open and willing way, wanting to talk about the events leading up to the offences and about her relationship to her previous partner. At this point in time, she accepted full responsibility for her actions, stating that she no longer blamed her ex-partner for her behaviour. This was in stark contrast to previous statements in which she firmly placed the blame for her actions on his shoulders. We wondered though if perhaps she realised that this change in thinking might improve her chances of getting custody of her baby.

The assessors took the assessment to their group supervision sessions during the six-week process and there the transference and countertransference experiences were discussed. The assessors felt a strong draw to collude with Bryony and Leo's wish for the assessors to gloss over the past. They wanted the assessors to remember the trauma that both of them had experienced as children, and more recently the trauma they experienced with the still birth of their first child. Bryony in particular wanted us to focus on the present situation that they were in and about their future plans, rather than her offences against the 12-year-old boy. When we pressed her to talk about what she had done to the boy it was apparent that Bryony believed a significant level of blame lay with Alex. There were times in the assessment when the assessors felt at odds with each other, believing that the other was possibly colluding and therefore unable to remain objective in the light of the strong feelings evoked by both parents. Similarly, the rest of the team who attended the supervision sessions felt very strongly that the assessors were siding with the parents, evidenced in a perceived tendency to minimise the risks and in highlighting the way that the system had let Bryony and Leo down when they were children.

At times the assessors felt frustrated, like they were 'losing their way' during the sessions. This also attested to the countertransference phenomena experienced with so many men or women who are both victims and perpetrators of sexual aggression. The job of the assessor – and when in treatment, the therapist – is to hold in mind the almost contradictory thoughts that this person has been severely traumatised and has traumatised others.

During the assessment period we were contacted by the lawyers who told us that Bryony and Leo had contacted social services who had then contacted the police regarding some comments posted on social media. Someone had posted a photo of a mother and a male child in a semi naked pose with the comment 'You wouldn't believe what she did – sicko bitch'. It seems likely that someone who knew about Bryony's past was trolling[2] her and had posted this image on her page. The police did not take the matter further and Bryony and Leo were encouraged to avoid social media.

During the assessment we noted that psychotherapeutic treatment had been recommended by professionals for both Bryony and Leo in the past but that so far this had not been made available. It was our opinion that the likelihood of reoffending would be reduced further if Bryony was to be referred to a suitable service able to provide trauma-focused forensic psychotherapy treatment.

The feelings evoked in us in the room ranged from disgust to a frustrating sense of not being able to reach Bryony. By the fourth session the assessment had taken on different qualities, and it felt as if Bryony was able to trust that the assessors were not going to criticise her for what she had done but instead that they were trying to understand with her how her actions had their roots in her experiences as a child. In their explanations the assessors hoped to instil in Bryony a sense of there being a common purpose. It became apparent that Bryony had some difficulties in fully taking in the impact of the violence and psychological abuse she had experienced at the hands of Alex. Similarly, the consequences of Bryony's experiences at the hands of her father were also out of her awareness and she spoke about feeling that her father's violence towards her was a way of her somehow protecting her mother from her father. I believe that without opportunities to process the trauma experienced by a violent aggressor, some clients are never able to understand the impact of their own violence on others.

Bryony talked about her childhood in a detached way, as she seemed to about most things. However, there were glimpses of sadness when she brought up her early experiences of being cared for. Bryony said she did not remember much about her early childhood, but she did say she remembered her father drinking heavily, beating up her mother and on at least one occasion he punched Bryony in the face. She also described a time when her mother left her in the street and so she went to her father's place of work and her father got angry with her for that. She also remembered throwing her belongings out of her bedroom window when she was angry and on a number of occasions she went missing but was not missed by her family.

Conclusion of the Risk Assessment

At the end of the process a comprehensive report was prepared that recommended, amongst other things, Bryony to attend weekly forensic psychotherapy. She had not been able to access any treatment while in prison due to there not having been any sex offender treatment programmes for women at that time. The level of risk was found to be medium given Bryony's understanding of the impact of her actions and the way she spoke about her offence. We also felt that with suitable treatment her risk to her baby, her other children and the wider community would probably reduce. The experience of being with her in the consulting rooms was one that oscillated between feeling confident that she was in a much better place psychologically than at any time previously, but also worrying that if things were to go wrong in her life she may fall into old patterns of behaviour. For instance, we were very concerned, that if her relationship with Leo ended then she may become more vulnerable and also riskier.

Bryony's experiences of being mothered and of mothering her first two children had left her numb to her own experiences of violence and in turn numb to her own sexual violence towards the neighbour's child. However, as she had not had any treatment in which she could start to process her own experiences, was it any wonder that Bryony did not seem to be able to process what she herself had done?

Due to her mother's experiences Bryony became a container for her mother's undigested trauma. The family home was not a nurturing and containing environment, with no support or encouragement available for Bryony to develop into a thoughtful and reflecting individual. Looking back through the family history the trauma did not simply start with Bryony's father. In attempting to find out more about the older generations it came to light that Bryony's grandmother had also been the victim of domestic violence.

Bryony was the receptacle of her father's domestic abuse and of her mother's neglect. Bryony's sadomasochistic relationship with Alex comes to represent her self-hatred of her own body. As Welldon (2011, p. 71) writes, this self-hatred perpetuates and reiterates the original abuse. Through a process of identification with her aggressors, Bryony then indirectly becomes the victimiser of her own children, through neglect or indifference, by 'choosing' to live with Alex when she might have been able to leave if she could.

In Court

About two months after the assessment was concluded there was a court hearing in the Family Court. Only one of the assessors was required to attend court on the day of the hearing and Bryony and Leo were keen to talk with the assessor before the hearing commenced. They attempted to ask the assessor why they had written some of the things they had and why they had made the recommendations they had. The assessor reinforced what they had been told about not being able to talk about these matters with them in the court. There was an agreement though to meet with them to go through the report once the proceedings were concluded. They were frustrated about this but accepted the offer to meet at another time. In the afternoon the judge called the assessor into the court in order to answer questions from the barristers about the content of the report.

A discussion of the unconscious processes that emerge and manifest themselves in the court room would take another chapter or book to discuss, but present in the court were the echoes of previous hearings in which Bryony lost custody of her children and in which she was convicted of her sexual crimes. They were ever present for her and for everyone in the room. Bryony became very tearful at times. Leo became angry and swore when the assessor was asked to back up comments in the report that questioned their ability to be good enough parents. Naturally, feelings burst out at times in the shape of looks and mutterings under their breath, but for the most part the couple kept a lid on their obvious anger and fear.

The assessor was able to provide the court with the evidence it needed to recommend a residential parenting assessment of Bryony, Leo and the baby. No decision was made concerning the possible return of Bryony's other children but the Sexual Harm Prevention Order was amended for the possible duration of the parenting assessment.

Conclusion

Although neither Bryony nor Leo had any discernible disability, I believe that the unprocessed trauma experienced by both of them increased the likelihood of them committing their varied offences. Bryony's sexual offences can be viewed as an externalisation of offences committed on her and the coercion and control that Alex had over her was significant. Leo's violence and drug related offences can also be seen as a result of not having had opportunities in which to process what was done to him as a child. Disability psychotherapy is useful here in helping us to think about the impact of trauma and its disabling impact.

Thinking about the impact of working with Bryony and Leo and of reading and hearing directly from them about their traumatic experiences, it is vital to take stock of the emotional and demanding nature of meeting people who are deeply traumatised, who have traumatised others. Keeping the tenets of disability psychotherapy in mind in these challenging clinical circumstances proved to be essential for the assessors in their efforts to stay focused and to think at a deep level about the complexities of court work, as well as the needs of the interested parties, all the while keeping the best interests of the children in mind.

As Corbett (2014) reminds us in risk and court assessment work:

> We are dealing here with patients who may be consciously seeking to minimise or deny their acts of abuse. They may also be unconsciously defended against our attempts to think with them about the impact on them of their disability, their relationships with their primary carers, or their experiences of loss and separation.

(p. 40)

We are often limited by the constraints of focusing our attention only on risk and the offences committed; we thereby miss the humanity and multifaceted, multi-dimensional nature of this work. The application of disability psychotherapy thinking is a significant aid in the pursuit of equality and justice for all.

Notes

1 All of the clinical material I describe has been carefully anonymised to protect confidentiality without losing the essence of the individual's situations and the associated dynamics.
2 Trolling is the act of leaving an insulting message on the internet in order to annoy someone.

Bibliography

Alvarez, A. (1992). *Live Company: Psychoanalytic Psychotherapy with Autistic, Borderline, Deprived and Abused Children.* London; New York: Routledge.

Corbett, A. (2014). Disabling Perversions: Forensic Psychotherapy with People with Intellectual Disabilities. *Forensic psychotherapy monograph series.* London: Karnac.

Corbett, A., Cottis, T. & Morris, S. B. (1996). *Witnessing, Nurturing, Protesting: Therapeutic Responses to Sexual Abuse of People with Learning Disabilities.* London: David Fulton.

Frankish, P. (2016) *Disability Psychotherapy: An Innovative Approach to Trauma-Informed Care.* London: Karnac Books.

Glasser, M. (1996). 'Aggression and sadism in the perversions' in Rosen, 2d edn, Oxford Medical Publications. Oxford, England; New York: Oxford University Press.

Kahr, B. (2002). *Forensic Psychotherapy and Psychopathology: Winicottian Perspectives* (The Forensic Psychotherapy Monograph Series). London: Karnac.

Kahr, B. (2020). *Dangerous Lunatics: Trauma, Criminality and Forensic Psychotherapy.* London: Confer Books.

Rosenfeld, H. (1971). 'A clinical approach to the psychoanalytic theory of the life and death instincts: an investigation into the aggressive aspects of narcissism.' *Int. J. Psychoanal.,* 52 (2): 169–178.

Sinason, V. (1992). *Mental Handicap and the Human Condition: New Approaches from the Tavistock.* London: Free Association Books.

Welldon, E. V. (1992). *Mother, Madonna, Whore: The Idealization and Denigration of Motherhood.* New York: Other Press.

Welldon, E.V. (2011). *Playing with Dynamite: A Personal Approach to the Psychoanalytic Understanding of Perversions, Violence, and Criminality. Forensic psychotherapy monograph series.* London: Karnac Books.

Chapter 6

The Respond Model of Disability Psychotherapy

The Attachment-Based Systems Approach

Noelle Blackman, Jess Lammin, Jasmine Hill, and Rosie Creer

The pioneering charity, Respond, was founded in 1991 by Tamsin Cottis, Steve Morris and Dr Alan Corbett. In 2003 Dr Noelle Blackman took up as Assistant Director, becoming CEO in 2012. Noelle and her co-authors were intrinsic to Respond's developing model of theory and practice until July 2023 and this chapter describes the therapeutic model that was in operation at Respond at that time. This chapter complements the contribution of other authors in this book who have also been part of this developing model.

This chapter will describe the model of disability psychotherapy that has developed over the last 30 years at Respond, a unique charity in the UK. Respond is a national charity; the vision is that all people with learning disabilities and autistic people who experience trauma are empowered to thrive. The mission as an organisation is that we reduce the impact of trauma in the lives of people with learning disabilities and autistic people, by developing trusting relationships through psychotherapeutically informed services.

There are a number of pioneering psychotherapists that have been both influential and supportive of Respond's work over the years. Tamsin Cottis, in her chapter in this book, specifically mentions Valerie Sinason whose concepts – The handicapped smile (Sinason, 1986) and Secondary Handicap (Sinason, 1992) – are central to our thinking. Another pioneer central to shaping the thinking and understanding of Respond's psychotherapists is Anne Alvarez, who has worked with us as a clinical supervisor for over 20 years. We have also been lucky enough to have Henrik Lynggaard as one of our clinical supervisors, whose systemic approach to working with people with learning disabilities is central to supporting the case management part of our psychotherapy model. It is the influence of these two supervisors that we will focus on particularly in this chapter.

It is important to set the scene regarding the way in which people with learning disabilities have been thought about historically.

The implementation of the National Health Service Act 1946 and the Mental Health Act (MHA) 1959 marked the beginning of the medicalisation of intellectual disability. Gates (2007) draws our attention to "…the strong emphasis in the definitions that was placed on treatment (within the MHA, 1959)" (p. 6). He adds "the Act made extensive reference to the Responsible Medical Officer. It is at this point

DOI: 10.4324/9781003646242-9

in the history of mental health legislation that the influence of medicine in defining the nature of learning disability exerted its greatest impact" (p. 6). With these two frameworks in mind, it is easy to understand why, up until the last few decades, people with learning disabilities have not had their emotional needs noticed; all symptoms have been responded to within a medical model of thinking. When emotional distress has been displayed as a change in behaviour the course of action has tended to be medication, cognitive behavioural therapy or a combination of the two. The aim has been to change the person's behavioural response rather than a more long-term aim of trying to understand and work with underlying distress or trauma (Blackman, 2012). Up until the last couple of decades there have rarely been many other options available.

In 1991 when Respond began we were a psychotherapy service that developed in response to the growing recognition that many people with learning disabilities had been sexually abused. We soon saw people who hurt others, recognising that they were often victims of abuse themselves. We also had a strong focus on changing the environment around the people we supported through providing training.

During the first decade of Respond there was a strong focus on highlighting how people with learning disabilities could benefit from the use of psycho-analytic psychotherapy. Up until this point there were only a few psy-chotherapy organisations (e.g. Tavistock clinic, St George's) or therapists (e.g. Professor Nigel Beail and Dr Pat Frankish) that made themselves accessible to this client group. The unfounded belief was that they would not be able to make use of this way of working (Bender, 1993). Psychotherapy is often con-sidered as a talking cure, however, as disability psychotherapists we have learned over the decades that it is far more profound than this. Psychotherapy is a relational process in which many forms of non-verbal communication take place and can be utilised as integral to the therapy.

What was learned at Respond over the first decade was the importance of making some changes within the usual way of providing psychotherapy. These changes are all linked to the fundamental elements that Corbett (2019) has highlighted as the foundations of disability psychotherapy. In particular attend-ing to the power imbalance between client and therapist, Corbett names this as holding respect for your client, as well as the importance of more warmth and less of a blank screen in the therapeutic relationship, and of bringing creative approaches to the work. Respond also recognises the trauma that comes with disability, particularly the two key aspects of clients' traumatogenic history described by Corbett "Firstly, disability is an intra and inter-psychic trauma. Secondly, societal responses to disability tend to exacerbate the primary trauma" (Corbett, 2019, p. 3). This is a constant awareness at the heart of the work.

In the year 2000 the Institute of Psychotherapy and Disability (IPD) was founded, amongst the clinicians who brought this to life were some of the psychotherapists from Respond. The IPD strives to describe, document and evidence a new development in psychotherapy.

Many of the current therapists working at Respond are arts psychotherapists; they may have trained as art therapists, drama therapists or dance and movement therapists, and some have gone on to further their training and done classic psychotherapy training as well. Some are classically trained psychotherapists who are creative in the way they work. All are able to build their therapeutic relationships with Respond clients using creativity.

Many of the people referred to Respond have experienced disproportionately high levels of deprivation, abuse and trauma beyond the primary trauma of disability. Thus a dynamic that can easily become triggered in therapy is one of victim and perpetrator. This dynamic can get into the therapeutic relationship and needs constant attention; it can also get into the whole organisation affecting relationships between Respond's staff. As a result, we are alive to it and work hard to attend to it through utilising externally facilitated monthly reflective practice sessions for the whole staff team.

Many clients who are referred to Respond have suffered early trauma within and from their families, however there are others who have supportive family who are actively involved in their everyday lives. The family are also likely to have experienced trauma through the fight to gain services and support for their child, which begins at first diagnosis and is lifelong. This can be seen as complex trauma which affects the whole family (Baker et al., 2021; Blackman et al., 2022,) the way in which they relate to one another and others around them and the way in which they can be perceived by others. This therefore makes it extremely important that all presenting symptoms are seen through a systemic and trauma-informed lens.

An in-depth awareness of the environment and culture in which the people referred to Respond are living is an important factor in informing the model that we have developed. Many clients rely on care workers and professionals in their everyday lives including to facilitate their attendance to therapy.

The Attachment-Based Systems Approach

Psychotherapy at Respond can offer the client with learning disabilities the chance to be understood through their entire communication. This takes place through: words and sounds, creative responses, body language and other non-verbal communication, and also countertransference. For people who find communicating through words difficult, being listened to in such a different way and being understood, perhaps for the first time, can be a profound experience.

Our model is informed by attachment theory, object relations theory, developmental theories, systemic theory and trauma theory, especially its impact on brain development and expression through the body (Blackman and Cottis, 2013). And as already stated creativity is at the heart of our approach.

From the early days of Respond the "advocacy" role that Tamsin mentions in her chapter has been a significant part of the way the organisation supports clients in therapy. It has felt impossible to provide therapy to someone with a learning disability or an autistic person without being aware of the injustice that they are experiencing on so many levels in their life outside of the consulting room.

Profound internal changes happen for a client during therapy; these take place through the new relational experience that psychotherapy can offer. The person often for the first time experiences a relationship where the power balance is considered and attended to, where someone is listening hard to all communication, verbal as well as non-verbal, to try to understand. Injustices are often voiced out loud and commented on by therapists, and this is often the first time a client will have experienced this. These changes are delicate vulnerable processes and it is too much to expect that the person will also have the ability to change the perception of others around them to their newly emerging self. Therefore, the "advocacy" or "case management" role has become increasingly important as a significant part of the therapy.

We believe that in order to bring about long-term change, the wider support network has to be in place and agree to become an integral part of the therapeutic process. In our experience, professionals and carers want to be given time to learn, reflect and share experience as they, like we, know that this can improve well-being and engender healthier relationships between people, so we work towards this as a part of the therapeutic approach.

From the earliest days of learning disability psychotherapy, the relationship between therapist, client and care network has been recognised as key (O'Driscoll, 2000). It is important to add that in the current climate of financially starved and target driven health and care services this can be a very real challenge to implement and maintain, but we have learned that this is imperative to the positive long-term outcome of the therapy.

All referrals that are accepted are recommended for a minimum of one year (44 sessions). Research has shown that defensive behaviour in people with learning disabilities will often stop within the first year of therapy (Carlsson et al., 2002). This has an important implication in the debate over why long-term therapy is often a better treatment model for people with learning disabilities; the fact is that it can take some time for long-term defences to come down, in order that deeper work can take place. Ending therapy too early can leave a client with learning disabilities in the vulnerable position of having recognised their defensive coping mechanisms and perhaps a feeling of having been "found out", but without any further work on ego strengthening or developing the ability to think (Blackman, 2012).

Each person starting therapy at Respond is assigned two therapists: they will have an individual therapist, with whom they meet weekly, and a second therapist – the "case manager therapist" who supports the systemic network. The case manager provides initial training to the client's support network and then becomes a bridge between this network and the confidential therapeutic work. Thus, the network becomes a tangible part of the transformative process of therapy as well as keeping the therapeutic relationship "safe".

The principles of systemic therapy are often applied in children's services and can be helpful to consider when working with people with learning disabilities who are also often dependent on others for support. The skills of the systemic therapist are noted as including the ability to influence conversations in a way that catalyses the strengths, wisdom and support of the wider system (Blackman and Cottis, 2013). This approach has been adapted by a number of therapists working with people with learning disabilities, notably Sandra Baum and Henrik Lynggaard (Baum and Lynggaard, 2006).

Transference and countertransference are core concepts of the psychodynamic and psychoanalytic approaches to psychotherapy and therefore integral to Respond's model.

Transference is the process by which a client displaces on to the therapist feelings which derive from earlier relationships. Countertransference means the conscious and unconscious reactions and feelings of the therapist to the client and to the transferred feelings of the client. The therapist uses her/his understanding of these feelings in order to work with the client. This is particularly important when working with people for whom talking is not their main way of communicating, as transference and countertransference are the main tools the therapist has with which to understand the thoughts and feelings of the patient and with which to bring about change.

In order for the therapist to be able to use countertransference it is essential that they can, as Hodges (2002) says "think about his or her own feelings and prejudices. Supervision and indeed personal therapy can make an essential difference in understanding the very complex emotional relationships created through our clinical work" (p. 26).

When working with a client with learning disabilities and who has very little speech, it can be the only tool one has for trying to understand their emotional state. It is to this which Hollins (1999) alludes when she states "Sometimes as clinicians we have to create hypotheses by observing and understanding human nature, but without diagnostic proof" (p. 7). The only "proof" we may have is the analysis of our own countertransferential feelings. It is important to consider that these unconscious processes are at play also within non-therapeutic relationships and in particular in the relationship between paid carer and client. Although of course these usually remain unconscious, it is important to raise the issue as it is the complex dynamic within this particular type of relationship which forms a key part of the "case management" within the Respond model.

Clinical Supervision As a Learning and Development Space for Respond Psychotherapists

Respond has a wonderful team of independent clinical supervisors who support our work and the continual development of our psychotherapists, with each of them bringing their rich experience and individual specialisms. They meet as a group with the Clinical Director quarterly, in order that there is a unified approach and thinking to the supervision and development needs across the organisation. They also contribute a clinical element to each therapist's annual appraisal. In this chapter we are focusing on just two of the supervisors, sharing two case studies that highlight their clinical work. The real names of clients are not used but permission to use their stories has been ethically granted and we have attempted to disguise any facts that might reveal their identity.

Working with the Unbearable

In supervision with Anne Alvarez, we are supported to consider the clinical work presented through some of the frameworks of understanding that she has developed over her career. One of these is the three different levels of psychotherapeutic work that Alvarez states are needed with dissociated or "damaged" patients (Alvarez, 2012, p. 10) in particular the third level that Alvarez writes about so powerfully in her book *Live Company* (1992), that of reclamation. She describes in a later work that "...*what* is being felt may, at certain moments, have to take precedence over *why* it is being felt, or even, on occasion, *who* is feeling it" (Alvarez, 2012, p. 3). We need to simply be with the client and have the ability to bear the feelings. This is so much easier said than done, whether the feelings are powerfully felt unconsciously or very live in the room. The temptation for the therapist may be to be make interpretations or ask questions when in fact this is the opposite of what is needed. Just being alongside in an undemanding way is not always easy – the feelings can be powerful and overwhelming – and gentle comments from the therapist on how this feels can be helpful, but not placing any further demands on the client is what is important.

Another presentation that we encounter with some of the people referred to Respond is that of seemingly hardly being present at all, being disassociated or closed down so much that it feels almost impossible to reach them. This can sometimes be hard to bear session after session. Alvarez (1992) describes this powerfully as a major experience in her work with psychotic children: "They seem to have gone beyond hope, memory and even fear ... there is nothing left on which to leave a trace, no imagined listener" (p. 13). In her work supervising our therapists at Respond, Alvarez enables us to find the glimmers of connection and thought and to build on them slowly and patiently. Having a supervisor who deeply understands this and can help to hold the hope needed has enabled us to see how important it is to be able to bear this for our clients.

Case Study by Jess Lammin

Donna, a young woman with a moderate learning disability was initially referred to an Independent Sexual Violence Advocate (ISVA) at Respond following multiple incidences of sexual assault. She was internally referred to Respond's Survivors Therapy Service and the referral was made during the COVID-19 pandemic to provide online therapy.

Donna was living in a supported living hostel for vulnerable people at the time and had been living there for two years. Donna had a good relationship with some of the staff at the hostel and felt well supported by her key worker, but also felt unsafe in the hostel as she had been sexually assaulted by one of the residents. Donna had been placed under a community mental health team (CMHT) and not in the learning disabilities team. Donna had also been diagnosed with Emotionally Unstable Personality Disorder (EUPD) and for several months after I started working with her, she was regularly admitted to A&E, on an almost weekly basis following serious incidences of self-harming (using a knife or razor, often on her arms but sometimes on her neck) or suicide attempts, usually by overdosing. None of these visits resulted in an inpatient admission or adequate follow-up and I was left feeling that neither she or her multiple attempts were being taken seriously. This was further played out by difficulties in communication with the care coordinator based in the CMHT and frequent cancelling of multi-disciplinary meetings or a repetition of the meetings being arranged on days when the case manager at Respond wasn't at work.

When I first met Donna, she seemed keen to talk and shared that she had never had any therapy, except for a short stint of counselling, aged 18, after her father passed away. Donna's grief was multiple and complex; her father had died of cancer and was the only relative who she felt had properly cared for her. Donna had experienced multiple losses of family members and more recently of her best friend the year before the COVID-19 pandemic hit. Donna had an estranged relationship with her sister, who she described as ignoring her calls and whose children she had never met, despite her continual attempts to make contact. Donna's grief was all consuming, she was fixated by the anniversaries of her loved-one's deaths and their birthdays as well as other milestones that she would obsessively ruminate over.

As well as multiple losses during childhood, Donna had been a witness to extreme domestic abuse and had experienced ongoing childhood sexual abuse. Having been abandoned by her mother as a baby and left with her father, she was brought up in an overcrowded and often volatile home with her paternal grandfather, maternal aunt and her husband, and later, her mother, new partner and her half, younger brother. Donna's older sister lived outside of the family home. Donna's first memory was at the age of two and a half years old where she witnessed eight police officers pulling her uncle off her aunt in a frenzied and prolonged attack that resulted in her aunt being hospitalised for several weeks.

Donna described how from the age of four, she had been collected every Sunday by her mother's cousin in his van, where he would take her to the nearby "scrubland" and sexually abuse her; this continued until she was 15 years old, when she realised that what was happening was not the experience of her peers and she finally got the confidence to tell her father. Despite her father being the one person that she felt loved by in her childhood and whom she idolised, he failed to report the abuse to the police, and she was left feeling that the abuse was her fault or even worse that he had been complicit. Donna was later able to get in touch with her rage at her father for his failure to protect her and this was especially hard for her as he was her main attachment figure.

Donna was bullied throughout her school life and by the time she was 16 she had dropped out of school entirely and had a new boyfriend. When her father died, she went to live at her boyfriend's mother's house and this relationship lasted for eight years but quickly became violent and abusive. The mother and sister were abusive too and Donna was told daily that she was ugly and stupid, so that by the time I met her these had become internalised scripts that she repeated about herself as well as experienced as external voices and intrusive commands telling her to hurt herself.

As well as hearing voices Donna experienced visual hallucinations which left her terrified at nighttime and meant that she had very disturbed sleep patterns, often not falling asleep until the early hours. Donna had learnt to manage the voices and hallucinations with alcohol which had developed into a dependency and was her only coping mechanism.

Whilst Donna had not had an official diagnosis of Complex Post Traumatic Stress Disorder (CPTSD), she was experiencing severe flashbacks and was extremely hypervigilant, living in constant fear for her life. This had not affected her ability to make relationships but the relationships she did have were unhealthy, abusive and controlling. Donna was bullied and harassed relentlessly by her peers and experienced severe hate crime throughout our work together. Several incidences were reported to the police, some of which were dropped, which added to her feeling of not being believed.

When I first met Donna, I was struck by her low sense of self-worth and strong feelings of not being good enough for anyone; she found it hard to think about her own needs, preferring to put others first. As is often the case with survivors of abuse there were strong feelings of shame and guilt around the abuse, but also associated were her feelings of rejection by her mother, who despite being in her life still was overly critical and emotionally withholding. Donna was depressed and anxious and had little hope for a better life.

However, despite this, Donna developed a good attachment to me and attended her therapy every week punctually, making good use of her sessions. During the start of therapy our work focused on her relationships, and she began to tell her life story by using a timeline that she worked on over several weeks. We thought about her trauma responses and how she had learnt to fawn, to make others happy as an adaptation to the abuse she had experienced and to survive. She worked using art to express her emotions and to think about what was important to her in a relationship and to begin to think about what she needed from others, rather than what they needed from her. This piece of work she revisited often.

At the end of each session Donna would often share things that she wanted to be communicated to the hostel staff, things that she felt unable to communicate herself. The case manager would act as a link person between her therapy and the hostel each week and vice versa. This way of joined up working allowed Donna to feel that I was still here, even when she wasn't with me. We came to an agreement that if she wanted to email me between sessions she could, but that I would read these before our next session for us to discuss in therapy. Eventually the emails became less frequent, and she became more able to communicate outside of sessions with the case manager so that we held the responsibility jointly, like a parental couple.

Donna's desire to harm herself usually came about when she was faced with painful feelings of separation, particularly when she was alone, which was when her voices would intensify and become more persecutory. Allen (as cited in Bateman & Fonagy, 2016, p. 88) has elaborated a complex model of trauma, defining it as "the experience of being left psychologically alone in unbearable emotional states". This could be seen in her insecure ambivalent attachment as there was the feeling she had never been securely held by her mother and she was reminded of this anxiety and pain whenever she was on her own. Respond needed to be that container (Bion 1962) for her to feel secure enough to hold herself in mind in her therapy and come to the slow realisation that others could also hold her in mind when she was not there.

The lack of holding by her mother was the origin of her split between her compliant and aggressive self, which would be seen when she felt that her care coordinator was not hearing her voice and she would become so dysregulated that she expressed fear that she would explode and attack staff in the hostel. For this same reason breaks were often experienced as overwhelming and early on in our work one break was felt so intensely that it put the therapy in jeopardy. The CMHT reacted by wanting to stop the therapy, feeling that it was triggering her self-harming and that her non-attendance after the break was a consent issue rather than Donna's distress about the break and her experience of it as an abandonment.

During breaks Donna would often increase her self-harming as a way to cope, which would be experienced by me on returning to therapy in the countertransference as guilt, fear and hopelessness that I wasn't and could never be enough. The case manager had to work carefully with the network to help them to think about the impact of breaks on Donna and how to mitigate her self-harming in the future.

Countertransferentially the repetition of unresponsiveness, as felt by Donna and staff working with her, by her care coordinator could be seen as a re-enactment of the care she had received as a child. This was in part due to her aunt, who was her main caregiver when her father was at work, having a diagnosis of paranoid schizophrenia and not always being able to provide the consistent care she needed. At times it would feel that there was a repetitiousness to the ongoing abuse that felt difficult to change in therapy and this sometimes caused a feeling of "stuckness" in the countertransference.

For therapy to be successful a secure attachment needed to be established, in which emotional states that were previously unbearable could be heard and made bearable, and through compassion and careful holding of the therapeutic space Donna was able to work through her grief, get in touch with difficult feelings of anger and shame and explore her feelings around her past trauma. She became better able to regulate her emotions, and was able to assert boundaries in her relationships, both professionally and personally. This in turn increased her self-esteem and enabled her to think about her future, moving on from the past trauma and focusing more on what she wanted her life to look like. About half way through the therapy she enrolled on a college course and was feeling more hopeful about her future. She had also begun to think about moving on from the hostel and the possibility of moving away from London and living by the seaside, which was a childhood memory she reminisced about, sitting on a beach with her dad, eating fish and chips.

Unfortunately, things started to unravel when she was bullied by men staying in a hotel next to the hostel, they took photographs of her coming and going to and from the hostel, made threats to harm her, including threats to rape and kill her. They sent her food deliveries and taxis multiple times a day so that she eventually became terrified to leave the hostel; this ultimately caused her to drop out of college and become very isolated.

Gradually Donna began to shift her view again. She was more able to look after herself and to explore the function of her self-harming and drinking. In supervision we thought about how, despite everything, she had survived so long and through so much, that there was a healthy part of her too. She began to make some new friends that seemed to be healthier relationships than those she'd had up until now and she started to be more independent. She visited new cities and developed new interests. She no longer focused obsessively on her grief, or the anniversaries of her loved ones. She built a resilience to the bullying and found relief in learning that meant she found it easier to ignore their constant messages on social media. Donna became better able to manage her strong emotions and stopped self-medicating through the daily drinking. By the time we had finished our work she had not been admitted to A&E for over a year and had not self-harmed as a way to manage for six months.

Clinical supervision supported me to think about how Donna's experience of being bombarded with violence since an early age had become a masochistic cycle, that she was always under attack and drawn into abusive situations and that this was a way for her to defend against traumatic events. Supervision was also key in working through my own anxieties around her risk of accidental death by cutting on her neck and arms, and my fear that the network, who were reactive and inadequate, were not going to keep her safe, repeating her parent's failures. In this way I had to hold the risk and notice what it was doing to me in the relationship. The supervisor and the supervision group thought with me about how Donna did not have much sense of self and had a critical super ego and how an important focus of the therapy was to support her in developing a stronger sense of herself through her experience of the therapeutic relationship. We also thought about how Donna often spoke in a way that was a defence rather than a communication and that sometimes this left my mind blank. We reflected that this was how she was feeling: empty and without thought. My supervisor encouraged me to slow the pace of the therapeutic work down, to enable us to really get hold of the loss she'd had in her life as well as to contain her emotional responses to this. Donna felt safe with me and experienced something new that she had not received before. Developmentally she related much earlier than her actual age, there was little symbolic thinking. It sometimes felt that there was a strong unconscious need to pass the trauma on (this was felt when she showed me sometimes graphic and very disturbing material that had been sent to her in text messages or on social media). We thought about how hard it was for Donna to hold onto the idea that I would believe her if I didn't witness the violence myself. It felt important that I knew something about how she felt. I was encouraged to show Donna that I knew and understood how bad she was feeling, to really validate her experiences, which sometimes meant I had to take up her rage and sense of injustice and fight for her, alongside her.

In supervision we thought about how her dependency on suffering was an addictive position and whilst it was so hard to get away from, we wondered what would be left if she did. Staying with feelings of desperation and hopelessness, it sometimes felt impossible imagining anything different than being a victim. We thought about her anger and how livid she was and that I could be furious too or help her to say no; how I needed to help her to stand up and say "enough", to support her to protect herself and for her to decide about how that was going to happen; and to help her to see that just because something is familiar, it doesn't mean that it is safe.

Donna was unable to come for the last few sessions and disengaged from her therapy after hearing that we would not get funding to extend beyond 18 months, having warned me several months before our ending that this was likely to happen. Donna had been able to share about other "healthy attachments" that she'd had in her life, including a mentor at school. Donna described that a part of them stayed inside her and that she carried them around with her and could imagine what they would say about things when life was difficult. I contacted her when she stopped coming to sessions to let her know that I thought it was too painful to have another ending, that it felt too difficult carrying on because she knew we were going to have to end and that perhaps it felt easier for her to leave me than to be left again.

I was able to pick up on how angry she was, and she could be angry with me in the transference; I could be the bad therapist for not getting funding for our work to continue, but good enough to stay around to the end. I wrote a therapeutic ending letter and in supervision we thought about how important it was to celebrate her achievements, to guard them, to make sure they were not lost.

The case management model acted as a container for Donna's intensely distressing feelings, experiencing the organisation as a holding place where she could be understood and things would be thought about and acted upon, which was a new experience for her. She felt taken seriously for the first time in her life. The case manager worked closely with the staff in the hostel who were caring and supportive, and she linked them up with the CMHT (who sadly remained laissez faire in their approach). However, it often felt that an invisible baton was being passed between myself, the case manager and the professional network or at least the hostel staff, that together we had created a net that would catch Donna if she fell. Over time she began to trust that process and to trust that the professionals around her had her back. This enabled her to grow stronger and begin to flourish.

Including the System As Part of the Therapeutic Process

As referred to earlier the relationships between therapist, client and care network are key to positive outcomes in disability psychotherapy. Corbett (2009) writes about the links between psychotherapy with people with learning disabilities and child psychotherapy:

> I would argue that both endeavours require the analyst to keep alive some memory, if not desire on behalf of the patient who, for cognitive and/or developmental reasons, does not keep it alive himself or herself. It is also a means of creating a parallel analytic process by which the surrogate parental figures are provided with their own space in which to think and reflect.
>
> (p. 48)

He goes on to suggest that as therapists we also need to assess the psychological capacity of the carers to support the analytic process. At Respond we would say that this is a key factor, as without the ability of the network to support the person in therapy, it is impossible/or very difficult to carry out the work. A key factor in the assessment process once referral for therapy has been made is whether the network is able and prepared to work with Respond to support the client in therapy. This is also why Respond therapy clients are allocated two psychotherapists – one who works directly with the person and the "case manager therapist" who works with the network.

In our supervision with Henrik Lynggaard the focus is on the work of our "case manager therapists". He describes the systemic process below:

> ... placing trust in the systemic process of opening space for dialogue and inviting all people in the room to have a voice (6 & 11) and by coordinating and exploring a multiplicity of views – that a relationally derived

knowledge gradually emerges from within the group of people who have convened. In other words, the creation of a relational space opens up relational possibilities and ways to go on, while placing heterogeneous perspectives in critical dialogue, can be highly generative.

(Lynggaard, 2017, pp. 45–46)

The case study below describes how we worked with someone referred to the Respond Transforming Care Service. This service supports people who have been subject to long-term hospital admissions to move back into their communities in a supportive and respectful way, in order that they successfully remain out of hospital. The model incorporates relational and therapeutic support directly to the person in hospital which begins as a relational circle as part of our adapted Circle of Support and Accountability (COSA) framework. Respond supports and collaborates with professionals within the multi-disciplinary team (MDT) throughout transition, from hospital to community and beyond, to ensure best possible outcomes. The main role of the circle is to model and successfully sustain healthy relationships with the person detained in hospital and to support them with holding the hope for a new life outside of hospital. Three members of Respond staff form each circle; gradually each member of the circle is introduced to the person and permission is sought from them prior to their commencement. Once all three members of the circle have been accepted, they take it in turns to offer 1–1 visits to the person whilst they are in hospital. These regular visits continue during the transition out of the hospital and last until the person becomes settled in their new home in the community. The three members of the circle work closely together. In their visits they spend time finding activities that the person enjoys and then these activities can be picked up and continued with any of the three circle workers. The experience of being supported in this way whilst in hospital means that the person begins to experience being "held in mind", building relationships with all three circle members who they experience as being linked up and consistent in their support of them. One of the circle workers is allocated a "lead" role, becoming the main contact from the circle with the person and the network both within and without the hospital. One of the three circle workers is a therapist and the role of the therapist within the circle is to support clinical thinking amongst the circle. The therapist can also at an appropriate point in time, having built some trust with them, support the person with understanding what psychotherapy is, how it might be helpful to them and how Respond can offer this.

Case Study by Jasmine Hill

Our work commenced with Lisa whilst she resided in hospital having been detained under Section 3 of the Mental Health Act (1983). Respond was commissioned to work with other professionals to support her in getting out of hospital and moving into a new home with a provider within the local community. The Respond team allocated to work alongside Lisa comprised of a case manager, three circle workers and a therapist.

Lisa is an adult in her 20s with mild intellectual disabilities who has experienced trauma throughout her childhood. It was reported that Lisa witnessed domestic violence between her parents and experienced physical and neglectful abuse within the family home. Lisa was known to social services from the age of four and was placed into foster care at the age of five following suspicious injuries.

Lisa experienced multiple foster and care placements all of which served notice due to her displaying behaviours that challenge. These included physical and verbal aggression towards herself but mainly towards others that cared for her. Lisa may have become attached to these historic behaviours and to being labelled or seen as "challenging", and identified with these reactive presentations which may have led her to believe that she was fundamentally unlovable.

Bowlby (1979, p. 365) stated that "humans especially infants rely on attachment figures for protection, comfort, and emotional regulation" and explored how the attachment forms between caregiver and baby set the foundations for future relationships. Davies and Frawley (1994) suggest that if the attachment bond is poor this is the most damaging psychological trauma. Schore (1994) emphasises that it is an attachment between caregiver and baby which is stored as a pattern for future experiences and relationships.

Mikulincer and Horesh (1999) draw attention to cases of parental neglect and rejection at a time of distress and need for support and how this could lead to the child developing an avoidant attachment style – one which is characterised by distrust, doubts regarding self-worth and chronic distress leading to social and emotional distancing and difficulties relying on others. Bartholomew, Henderson and Dutton (2001) declare that individuals who may have experienced inconsistent and insensitive parenting may seek the desire to form close relationships in search of a secure base but present with conflicting emotions, fearing rejection and seeking control. In adulthood this might result in an anxious-avoidant attachment style whereby the individual simultaneously has positive and negative perceptions of others (Ainsworth, Blehar, Waters and Wall, 1978). The period in Lisa's life when she was detained in hospital resulted in her experiencing an everchanging support team who would swap shifts every hour. This pattern may have had a significant impact on the opportunities available for Lisa to develop connections and form relationships with her support staff which could reinforce the insecure attachment style and anxious avoidant tendencies she had developed as an infant.

Due to Lisa's anxious-avoidant tendencies as a result of experiencing early relational trauma, my role as a circle worker was to develop a relationship with Lisa where she felt heard, contained and safe; a relationship which modelled clear boundaries, empathy and provided her with a consistent approach and attunement.

Within Respond's "Transforming Care" framework, the lead circle worker had established a good rapport with Lisa whilst she resided in hospital. This enabled us to introduce another circle worker. I was introduced using a one-page profile. This included information about me to allow Lisa to familiarise herself with me through sharing my likes and dislikes, hobbies and interests, and why I work for Respond. Through sharing my one-page profile, Lisa was able to form connections through shared interests which encouraged her to speak with me. Our initial contact was sporadic and occurred through text messages and brief phone calls. Gearity (1996, p. 72) proclaimed that a secure attachment is developed from two main elements. The first of these is the establishment of a basic sense of trust in the world: "When I need you, you will be there" (Gearity, 1996). This basic sense of trust was established through my consistent availability. Although there were some boundaries in terms of the days and hours Lisa could speak with me, I ensured that whenever Lisa called or contacted me, I made sure I would respond within a relatively short time frame. Thus, I enabled Lisa to start to develop a sense of trust in our relationship, seeing me as someone who is available, responsive and helpful should adverse or stressful situations arise (Karen, 1994).

The second element which Gearity (1996) addresses is the allowance for emotional regulation, including the expression of feelings. These set the foundation for a secure attachment in future relationships. Through establishing a basic sense of trust with Lisa she was able to manage pre-arranged weekly phone calls with me and would rarely call outside of these times, which suggests that Lisa felt contained and safe within our relationship and trusted that our contact would be regularly maintained.

Following months of planned and consistent contact through arranged telephone and text conversations, Lisa expressed that she felt safe enough to meet with me in person. Unfortunately, it was also during this time that the COVID-19 pandemic occurred which led to the hospital cancelling all visitors on the ward. To overcome this obstacle and continue to build rapport, we planned regular contact in the form of video calls. Due to the restrictions in place, I was not able to meet Lisa in person until after she had transitioned out of hospital. Lisa experienced consistency regarding her support staffing team in her new community placement; this increased her prospects to develop healthy attachments and form connections towards her regular support staff.

Although our relationship remained consistent throughout Lisa's transition, it was not without its challenges. Due to Lisa's avoidant and anxious characteristics, she would often cancel our visits but then seek connection through multiple telephone calls across her team at Respond. It was through systemic supervision I was able to explore what Lisa was communicating; not only through her verbal communication, but also through what was not being spoken but acted out through cancelling visits. Systemic supervision highlighted that Lisa was presenting with a desire to form a close relationship but simultaneously a fear of being rejected. Lisa's defence mechanisms seemed to be actively maintaining her anxious-avoidant attachment style, perhaps to keep herself safe (Baum and Lynggaard, 2006).

Bowlby (1980) draws attention to the relationship between attachment and defences, declaring that these defence mechanisms first develop in childhood when the caregiver's response to their child's fear or distress is inadequate, thus implying that individuals who are insecurely attached display defence mechanisms to a greater extent. This stressed the importance of consistency within my approach, whilst also allowing flexibility within the boundaries to enable Lisa to make contact and seek connection through telephone calls and rearranged visits. In other words, to enable our relationship to continue, it was essential that I allowed the social interactions to be on Lisa's terms for us then to develop a framework to work within (Case and Dalley, 1993).

What we particularly value about the systemic approach is its focus on context, relationships, communication and interaction; that is, what is happening between people rather than within people, since this moves us away from pathologising individuals and towards viewing concerns and problems as interpersonal.

This reinforced that working collaboratively not only with the individual, but her wider support network was crucial. It was important that Respond did not come across as the outsider expert, but instead as one group of people who were seeking to co-ordinate and work collaboratively in the best interests of Lisa. Respond joined the network in the "not-knowing position" (Anderson 1995, p. 30), that is, not knowing in advance what would be best for Lisa and creating room for different types of expertise, including Lisa's voice. In practical terms we arranged network meetings which included Lisa and Respond and offered reflective practice for her support staff including the management. Instead of focusing solely on Lisa's patterns of behaviour or her "acting out", we also explored the non-verbal communication and the meanings these may hold. Shotter (1993, pp. 102–103) introduced the term "relational knowing", or "knowing with", that is a knowledge that develops and emerges through interaction with others. It was this "knowing with" stance which helped to engage other practitioners in collaborative working and which enabled boundaries and a framework to be established. Working systemically also enabled us to consider the beliefs, attitudes and expectations of the relational role for the circle workers.

For 18-months, Lisa and I worked together in a relational capacity. Our circle visits occurred mostly every three weeks and our telephone calls were contained to once a week. My circle visits took place at Lisa's home in the community. I sought to further develop my rapport with Lisa by joining her in practical tasks of her choosing. During, my visits, we would usually bake cakes and engage in art activities linked to events which Lisa celebrated. I found that by working alongside Lisa on a practical task she was able to tell me about what was important in her life which gave us the opportunity to explore how she was feeling. This suggested that the relationship we had established was what Winnicott (2005, pp. 63–64, 150, 176) would term "good enough".

Through discussion in systemic supervision, collectively the team recognised the many achievements which Lisa had accomplished since leaving hospital and the idea of proposing a reflective journal for Lisa to complete was suggested. Lisa's journal became a key element to each circle visit as it contained entries about her goals, milestones and achievements since her engagement with Respond.

It was towards the end of my relational involvement when Lisa expressed a desire to re-engage with Respond's therapy service. Lisa had previously attended a few assessment sessions but then requested for these assessments to be placed on hold and eventually Lisa decided that she no longer wished to engage which ended the assessment period. Lisa's request to re-engage with therapy posed a dilemma for the team at Respond in terms of assigning a therapist who had capacity. After much discussion in both clinical and systemic supervision, a decision was made to propose to Lisa that I could offer to see her in my other capacity as therapist at Respond. This change was possible as my role as Lisa's circle worker was reaching its agreed end. Within Respond's "Transforming Care" framework, 18 months marks the timeframe where the third circle worker would end working with an individual.

When proposing this transition to Lisa and her wider support network, it was important that we highlighted that I would naturally be ending my circle work due to the 18-month time limit. However, this opened the opportunity for me to offer to transition into becoming her therapist. Lisa gave her consent for this transition stating, *"I'm so happy Jasmine is going to be my new therapist, I thought I would have to get to know someone new, but I've got Jasmine. Thank you so much".* It seemed to the team that the process of investing time in accompanying Lisa from hospital to community and gradually building a trusting relationship, through texts, telephone calls, visits and engagement in shared tasks, had shown that more solid connections could become established. That is, social connections were established that were not destined to succumb to repeating patterns of rejections and rupture.

In order to facilitate the explanation of the change in my role from circle worker to Lisa's therapist, I used easy read information with Lisa to describe what an art therapy session could look like and what the term "therapy" means. Using easy to read language supported by pictures enabled Lisa to process and reflect on the change of dynamics within our relationship and to familiarise herself with what our therapeutic relationship could look like in terms of the different boundaries and framework and how these may differ from our circle work. This enabled a smooth transition from my role as circle worker to Lisa's therapist. As part of Lisa's journey into therapy, she came for an initial visit to the Respond clinic. Through this visit Lisa was able to become familiar with the journey to therapy, the setting and the therapy room, so that when her therapy commenced this would be somewhere recognisable to her and help to minimise her anxieties.

In conclusion, through working collaboratively with the individual, her wider support network and through systemic supervision the team at Respond was able to successfully provide consistent support to an individual with mild intellectual disabilities to transition out of hospital and into a provider within the community. This provided Lisa with continuity in terms of her care and support. It was through working collaboratively that I was able to offer a smooth transition from working with Lisa in a relational capacity to becoming her one-to-one therapist to support her with life in the community. This transition was able to take place due to establishing a base sense of trust within my circle role with Lisa, which took 18 months to develop.

The Importance of Reflective Practice As a Way of Managing Trauma Disturbing the Healthy Functioning of the Organisation

Organisations which work with traumatised and/or disabled clients may be vulnerable in particular ways (Hopper 2012). Society's view that people with learning disabilities have little or no worth, or are a drain on resources (Curen 2013) and will never "get better", may find its way into the fabric of the organisation. This may affect staff morale or lead to a sense of fragility in the purpose of the organisation. Hopper describes how organisations engaged in trauma-based work have a tendency to cohere or fragment in way which may damage organisational structures. Healthy difference between colleagues may be difficult to foster. Respond is alive to this vulnerability in its own functioning. It also recognises that the organisations with whom it works – either in its work with members of the client's network, or in its broader services – will be vulnerable to these dynamics too. They will impact on the client, and the network, and, as such, they are relevant to our clinical model (Blackman and Cottis, 2013).

Conclusion

Respond have developed a creative, relational model of psychodynamic psychotherapy with traumatised autistic and learning disabled clients that includes a systemic approach. Our findings are that the therapy needs to be long term for a minimum of one year. A key factor in the work is to "be alongside" the client and to be aware of and attend to the unconscious power dynamic in the therapeutic relationship. We have learned that within the attachment-based systems model it is important for long term successful outcomes to have two therapists for each client: one who works directly with the client and one who works with the support network, the "case manager therapist". Their role is to enlist the support of the network around the client in support of the change that all are working towards with the client. It is an integral part of achieving this change.

Bibliography

Ainsworth, M. D. S., Blehar, M. C., Waters, E., and Wall, S. (1978). *Patterns of Attachment: A Psychological Study of the Strange Situation.* Hillsdale, NJ: Erlbaum.

Allen, J. G. (2004). *Coping with Trauma: A Guide to Self-Understanding* (2nd edn). Washington DC: American Psychiatric Press.

Allen, J. G. (2012). *Restoring Mentalizing in Attachment Relationships: Treating Trauma with Plain Old Therapy.* Washington DC: American Psychiatric Press.

Allen, J. G. (2013). *Mentalizing in the Development and Treatment of Attachment Trauma.* London, UK: Routledge.

Alvarez, A. (1992). *Live Company; Psychoanalytic Psychotherapy with Autistic,* Borderline, Deprived and Abused Children. London and New York: Routledge.

Alvarez, A. (2012). *The Thinking Heart; Three levels of psychoanalytic therapy with disturbed children.* London and New York: Routledge.

Anderson, H. (1995). Collaborative language systems: Towards a post-modern therapy. In R. Mikeshell, D. Lusterman, & S. McDaniel (Eds), *Integrating Family Therapy: Handbook of Family Psychology and Systems Theory* (pp. 27–44). Washington, DC: American Psychiatric Association.

Baker, P., Cooper, V., Tsang, W., Garnett, I. & Blackman, N. (2021). A survey of complex trauma in families who have children and adults who have a learning disability and/or autism. *Advances in Mental Health and Intellectual Disabilities, 15*(5), 222–239. Emerald Publishing Limited.

Bartholomew, K., Henderson, A. J. Z. and Dutton, D. G. (2001). Insecure attachment and abusive intimate relationships. In C. Clulow (Ed.), Adult Attachment and Couple Work: Applying the 'Secure Base' Concept in Research and Practice (pp. 43–61). London, England: Routledge.

Bateman, A. and Holmes, J. (1995). *Introduction to Psychoanalysis Contemporary Theory and Practice.* London: Routledge.

Bateman, B. & Fonagy, P. (2016) *Based Treatment for Personality Disorders: A Practical Guide* (p. 88). Oxford: Oxford University Press.

Baum, S. & Lynggaard, H. (2006). *Intellectual Disabilities: A Systemic Approach.* London: Karnac.

Bender, M. (1993). The Unoffered Chair: The History of Therapeutic Disdain towards People with a Learning Difficulty. *Clinical Psychology Forum, 54,* 7–12.

Bion, W. (1962). *Learning from Experience,* London: Karnac Books.

Blackman, N., (2012). *The Use of Psychotherapy in Supporting People with Intellectual Disabilities who have Experienced Bereavement.* Unpublished PhD dissertation. University Herts.

Blackman, N. and Cottis, T. (2013). *Psychotherapy at Respond: The Relational and Attachment-Based Systems Model.* Unpublished.

Blackman, N., Vlachakis, K., Annes, A., Griffin, S. & Baker, P. (2022). Brief report on six clinical cases of trauma in families that have children and adults who have a learning disability and/or are autistic. *Tizard Learning Disability Review, 27*(2), 69–77.

Bowlby, J. (1979). *The Making and Breaking of Affectional Bonds.* London and New York: Routledge.

Bowlby, J. (1980). *Attachment and Loss: Vol. 3. Loss.* New York, NY: Basic Books.

Carlsson, B., Hollins, S., Nilsson, A. and Sinason, V. (2002). Preliminary findings: an Anglo-Swedish psychoanalytic psychotherapy outcome study using PORT and DMT. *Tizard Learning Disability Review, 7(4)*, 39–48.

Case, C. and Dalley, T. (1993). *The Handbook of Art Therapy.* London and New York: Routledge.

Circles of Support and Accountability (COSA) UK. https://circles-uk.org.uk/.

Corbett, A. (2009). Words as a second language: The psychotherapeutic challenge of severe intellectual disability. In T. Cottis (Ed.), Intellectual Disability, Trauma and Psychotherapy (pp. 45–62). London: Routledge.

Corbett., A. (Ed.) (2019). *Intellectual Disability and Psychotherapy: The Theories, Practice and Influence of Valerie Sinason.* London and New York: Routledge.

Curen, R. (2013). Laying the ghosts to rest: a therapeutic approach to the treatment of a sexually abused man with a learning disability. *The Psychotherapist, 53*, 10–12.

Davies, J. M. and Frawley, M. G. (1994). *Treating the Adult Survivor of Childhood Sexual Abuse: A Psychoanalytic Perspective.* New York: Basic Books.

Gates, B. (2007). *The Nature of Learning Disabilities.* In B. Gates (Ed.) Learning Disabilities: Towards Inclusion (5th Edition). London: Elsevier.

Gearity, A. (1996) *Attachment theory and real life: How to make ideas work.* Accessed from: http://education.umn.edu/ceed/publications/early%20report/spring96

Hodges, S. (2002). *Counselling People with Learning Disabilities.* London: Palgrave.

Hollins, S. (1999). Developmental Psychiatry – Insights from Learning Disability. Paper presented at the Blake Marsh Lecture at the Annual Meeting of the Royal College of Psychiatrists, Birmingham.

Hopper, E. (2012). (ed.). *Trauma and Organizations.* London: Karnac.

Karen, R. (1994). *Becoming Attached: First Relationships and How They Shape Our Capacity to Love.* Oxford: Oxford University Press.

Lynggaard, H E., (2017). *Learning Disabilities and Systemic Psychotherapy: A Field of Rich Learnings.* Doctoral thesis, Department of Critical Disability Studies and Psychology. Manchester Metropolitan University.

Mental Health Act. (1983). Section 3. Government of the United Kingdom. Accessed from https://www.legislation.gov.uk/ukpga/1983/20/contents

Mikulincer, M. & Horesh, N. (1999). Adult attachment style and the perception of others: The role of projective mechanism. *Journal of Personality and Social Psychology, 76(6)*, 1022–1034. *Doi: 10.1037/0022–3514.76.6.1022.*

National Health Service Act. (1946). *Parliamentary Archives,* HL/PO/PU/1/1946/ 9&10G6c81. Accessed from https://www.legislation.gov.uk/ukpga/1946/81/pdfs/ukp ga_19460081_en.pdf

O'Driscoll, D. (2000). *'Do the feebleminded have an emotional life?' A history of psychotherapy and people with learning disabilities.* Unpublished master's dissertation. Regents College, London.

Schore, A. (1994). *Affect Regulation and the Origin of the Self: The Neurobiology of Emotional Development.* Mahwah, NJ and Hove: Lawrence Erlbaum.

Shotter, J. (1993). *Conversational Realities: Constructing Life through Language.* London: Sage.

Sinason, V. (1986). Secondary Mental Handicap and its relationship to trauma. *Psychoanalytic Psychotherapy 2*(2), 131–154.

Sinason, V. (1992). *Mental Handicap and the Human Condition.* London: Free Association Books Ltd.

UK Mental Health Act. (1959). Accessed from https://shorturl.at/hturC

Winnicott, D. (2005). *Playing and Reality.* London & New York: Routledge Classics.

Chapter 7

From Trauma to Creative Integration

Disability Psychotherapy and the Evolution of a Systemic Model of Trauma Treatment for Vulnerable Children and Adults

Eimir McGrath

It all started from a rather sudden, unanticipated shift into disability psychotherapy following a hiatus in my working life. Over the previous 25 years and with a background in psychology and Montessori teaching, I had taken on varied roles: working in infant and early childhood research, therapeutic work with children and adolescents in residential settings, teaching from preschool to postgraduate level, and working with refugee and asylum seeker children and their parents in a socially deprived area of Dublin's inner city. Throughout these years, I also taught ballet and Laban community dance.

I was between jobs, an opportunity had arisen to undertake an MA in Dance and together with serendipitously spotting an advertisement in a local newspaper for a play therapist, the future started to take on an unexpected shape. The play therapy post came with funding to access postgraduate training, which eventually evolved into a qualification in both child and adult psychotherapy. I had acquired a post where psychotherapy was a novel addition to a very medicalised model of care, in an institutional setting that provided a home for a group of children and adults with multiple disabilities. Over the next few years, I began to explore the world of disability from both a clinical and an academic perspective, with MA studies developing into a transdisciplinary PhD (McGrath, 2013) that combined dance, critical disability studies, attachment theory and the neurobiology of relationship.

Out of this melting pot of learning and experiencing, a systemic model of trauma treatment developed that has relevance in multiple settings, with a focus on vulnerable children and adults who often require support services. Tracing this pathway over the past two decades is a daunting task, as there were so many twists and turns that led me in so many unexpected directions. In trying to find a coherent way to explore all these elements for the purpose of this chapter, I found my focus in thinking about three internationally renowned psychotherapists who have not only had a profound effect on my development as a disability psychotherapist, but also fundamentally

DOI: 10.4324/9781003646242-10

contributed to the development of my clinical practice for children and adults without disabilities who have experienced sexual abuse, complex trauma and dissociative disorders.

Firstly, Dr. Valerie Sinason's seminal text *Mental Handicap and the Human Condition* (Sinason, 2010 [1992]) gave me a psychoanalytic insight into all that I was experiencing in my early days of working with children and adults with multiple disabilities. In that maelstrom of institutionalised life, of behaviourally driven interventions and organisational lack of therapeutic thinking, discovering this book was like a beacon of light that gave me hope and direction in the creation of a psychotherapeutic service where none had existed previously. Her concepts such as the handicapping process, primary and secondary handicap, the handicapped smile and disability as a defence against trauma (Sinason 2010) all gave shape and meaning to the rather chaotic and confusing interactions with both staff and residents that until then did not hold any real coherence of understanding for me. The constant directives by staff to the residents to smile in order to replace any expression of anxiety or distress; the insistence that the visibly angry young man I was introduced to was 'very contented, except when he spits at you', suddenly made sense when I read:

> Guilt that people exist who have to bear unfair and appalling emotional, physical or mental burdens can be so unbearable that a state of denial is brought about where those in greatest pain are asked to be the happiest.
> (Sinason, 2010, p. 119)

Discovering this book and the onward directions in which it sent me, provided a secure and inspiring theoretical base upon which to explore, reflect and integrate learning and practice in my clinical work. I am extremely fortunate and very thankful to still have Valerie's deep humanity, wisdom and immense knowledge to call upon in person, as she continues to play an integral part in my professional life as my clinical supervisor.

As my work progressed, I started receiving referrals for children on the autistic spectrum with highly complex needs, who tended to arrive at my door as a last resort. These children had often already experienced a very high level of psychological and behavioural supports and interventions that did not appear to have reduced their distress and disconnection from the world around them. As there was (and unfortunately often still is) a widely held misconception that people with disabilities do not have the facility to engage fully in a psychotherapeutic relationship, I was the final point of contact in seeking help when all else seemed to be failing. Another book came to my rescue in trying to find a theoretical underpinning for working with these 'hard to reach' children. Dr. Anne Alvarez's *Live Company* (1992) provided me with a deep, psychoanalytical understanding of the path to connectedness with children who experience a disintegrated, or even unintegrated way of being in the world. Her approach to working with such children was further developed in *The Thinking Heart* (2012) and her exploration of three levels of connectedness, from vitalising the other at the most primitive level, through the descriptive amplification of the other's affective states, to the capacity for thinking and symbol formation within relationship with one another provided me with a blueprint for exploring meaning within the intersubjective happenings in the therapy room. The application of this theoretical thinking to adults who often arrived to me with a dual diagnosis of intellectual disability and autism, gave me a deeper understanding of the non-verbal, unconscious processes at play within these therapeutic relationships. I have the wonderful privilege of having a supervisory relationship in recent years with Anne where I can continue to learn from her exceptional insight and expertise.

The third person who had a profound effect on my development as a psychotherapist was the late Dr. Alan Corbett. His untimely death in 2016 was an enormous loss for the psychotherapy world, particularly those of us practising disability psychotherapy, but his legacy lives on in his many published works, including his most recent books (Corbett, 2014, 2016), which provide such rich insight, scholarship and depth of clinical thinking. This chapter was originally to be written for a book as part of a series edited by Alan, exploring the ways in which mainstream psychotherapy is enriched by the learning contained in disability psychotherapy. Sadly, it was an unfinished project which for me is now coming to fruition as I reflect here on how starting a psychotherapy practice with some of the most vulnerable and disenfranchised members of our society has enabled me to develop relational, communicative and creative ways of connecting with anyone who may not otherwise feel, or be considered, reachable in the more traditional psychotherapeutic tradition of the 'talking cure'.

I also found Alan through a book. As my work progressed in the field of disability, I was faced with the constant presence of not only disability trauma (Sinason, 2002, 2010), but also complex trauma and sexual abuse, and I sought out anything in print that might inform my practice. *Witnessing, Nurturing, Protesting: Therapeutic Responses to Sexual Abuse of People with Learning Disabilities* (Corbett, Cottis and Morris, 1996) came out of the work of Respond[1] where Alan was a founder director. I was acutely aware of the need for specialist clinical supervision and having read this book, I tracked down contact details and introduced myself to him by email. To my enormous relief and delight, I discovered that he was available for clinical supervision in Dublin and so our relationship began, which continued right up until his death. His deep curiosity that was seated in huge empathy and compassion, along with his rich clinical insight in the face of intra- and interpsychic pain, organisational struggles and systemic failings, shaped my practice in the most fundamental ways. His mentorship, collegiality and friendship supported and guided me throughout these years. With all three supervising psychotherapists, I am struck by the pathway from a disembodied, cerebral connection through a book, to relationship, the bedrock of all therapeutic work. It is this power of the relationship that makes therapeutic connection and change possible (Schore, 2019), regardless of the intellectual capacity of the client (Corbett, 2009; Sinason, 2010).

Alan Corbett's synopsis of the fundamental aspects informing the core ethos of disability psychotherapy (Corbett, 2019, p. 2) encapsulates the development of my clinical work. He wrote of six aspects: awareness of cultural issues, respect, trauma, boundaries, the unconscious, and creativity. I will trace my path from the beginning of my practice to the present day by weaving these together in a chronology of my own growth as I first wrestled with the notion of disability in societal terms; as I became aware of the fundamental role of respect in setting up a disability psychotherapy service; and as I faced the depth of trauma inherent in this work and refined a treatment approach grounded in intersubjectivity and creativity.

The Sociocultural Concept of Disability

Living with a disability in contemporary western society inherently means living within a system that discriminates against, and excludes to varying degrees, all those whose bodies and minds do not fit within the accepted notion of normative functioning (Snyder and Mitchell, 2006; Garland-Thomson, 2009; McGrath, 2012). This is the lived reality of disability. What should be experienced as a shared interdependence and an acceptance of vulnerability between all members of a community, often becomes a disempowering experience with disability being perceived as deficit and loss, rather than an alternative way of being.

Bill Hughes, disability scholar and activist, discusses the notion of ableism[2] and the process of social exclusion. He states:

> ... ableism makes the world alien to disabled bodies, and, at the same time, produces impairment as an invalidating experience. It is manifest in our cultural inclination towards normalcy by way of correction, towards homogeneity by way of disparagement of difference.
>
> (Hughes, 2012, p. 24)

The residential centre where I began my psychotherapy journey was very much a product of mid-twentieth century approaches to the care of the intellectually disabled and reflected Hughes' statement regarding ableism. Many of the older adult residents had been placed into care as infants, their disabilities beyond the possibility of 'correction', and so far beyond 'homogeneity' (Hughes, 2012, p. 24), that the societally prescribed solution of institutionalisation was imposed on parents as being the best, if not only, option for both them and their child. This institutionalisation of those considered abnormal, philosopher Michel Foucault's 'carceral archipelago' (1991, p. 6), was designed to normalise a population where:

' ... the supervision of normality was firmly encased in a medicine or a psychiatry that provided a sort of "scientificity"; it was supported by a judicial apparatus which, directly or indirectly, gave it legal justification' (Foucault, 1991, p. 296).

This is the carceral history of the majority of the older adults who have been referred to me, one which we all hold within the communal psyche. A few residents had the continuity of a loving family connection; others had been effectively abandoned apart from an annual visit from family, by invitation, to attend a religious service for the 'blessing of the sick'. This was one of my first experiences of the power of the communal psyche to uphold an ableist notion of sickness contained in disability, and the consequent disempowerment of the disabled person it contains. Up until the changes brought about in the early 2000s, monies rightfully belonging to the older residents that could have been used to enhance their lives were put into individual funeral funds so that they carried the cost of their own deaths. The possibility of enhanced lived experiences was superseded by the need to offset the expenses of disposing of those 'disposable bodies' (Goodley, Lawthom and Runswick, 2014). This expression of the annihilatory fear held within disability (Sinason, 2020, p. 58), a life not worth living by normative standards, was starkly enacted in this scenario.

When disability is considered as a social construction, it uncovers the existence of negating learned responses that are expressed possibly as an uncomfortable sympathy coupled with a patronising admiration, imagining an ongoing struggle for survival as a result of the burden of being disabled; or by infantilising those with an intellectual disability as 'wondrous permanent children who inhabit a Never Never Land where sexuality will never intrude' (Sinason, 2010, p. 23). Sometimes an even greater degree of admiration is extended to the carers of those with disabilities, who are perceived to bear the burden, reflecting an understanding of disability that is based on deficit and suffering, an inherently medical interpretation of embodied difference as 'abnormal' (Longmore, 2009, 143).

I was also acutely aware of the communal responses to disability based on a combination of not only pity, but also at times an underlying fear and need for avoidance. This can be a reflexive reaction related to a primordial emotional response of fear and disgust that identifies difference as threatening (Cozolino, 2017, p. 288). The connected phenomena of hypervisibility/invisibility of those whose being in the world is perceived as abnormal, triggers the shaming stare or the dehumanising averted gaze of those who wish to defend against the acceptance of vulnerability that is part of the human condition (Garland-Thomson, 2009; Hughes, 2012, p. 25; McGrath, 2019, p. 23).

In my early days at the residential centre, I frequently had to confront my own inherent prejudice, fear and disgust as I struggled with smells, sights and sounds that were unfamiliar and unsettling. My first introduction to the adult group was at breakfast time, where all were gathered in one room to be fed.

The visual impact was enormous, I had never seen such concentrated embodied diversity and I was immediately reminded of philosopher Mikhail Bakhtin's (1984) notion of Rabelaisian carnival and the grotesque, where the disorganised, disabled body that lacks control evokes the realisation, and consequently the fear, that this embodiment is a possibility for everyone. Some level of infirmity is a certainty, regardless of how much control each person perceives to have over his or her current state of being (McGrath, 2013), not only in body, but also in mind, when facing disability may touch 'on the terror we hold in our unconscious about losing our own capacity to think' (Corbett, 2014, p. 4).

I became acutely aware that in order to work in this field, societally pre-scribed and preconceived notions of disability needed to be explored and challenged so that therapeutic relationships can be formed that are fully open to the humanity of the other.

As I slowly adjusted to this new milieu, the personhood of each individual began to shine through. I started individual therapy sessions after successfully negotiating and declining the request from a senior member of staff that several other residents could perhaps watch, lined up in their wheelchairs along the sides of the therapy room. One of my first clients was Steven, the angry young man who had no words, but could spit over impressive distances with amazing accuracy. He was delivered to my room in his wheelchair, very obviously against his will and with a mask dangling from a handle, with the instruction that I was to place it over his mouth whenever he was about to use this form of communication. I was alarmed, concerned for the care worker who was obviously anxious at being given this task of Steven's delivery, and even more concerned by my proximity as a very justifiable target. I welcomed Steven to the room and immediately told him that there are two important things for him to know: he's the boss of choosing to come into this room to spend time with me, and, I will never put a mask over his mouth when he needs to spit. He stared at me for several seconds that felt interminable and then turned his head away, but did not spit.

Respect

Steven's entry into my therapy room exemplified many of the difficulties facing people with disabilities in their everyday lives. Autonomy and agency are often compromised as each disabled person is within a system of care over which they have very little control. Their lives are part of a complex relational system where care workers in both residential and daycare settings often take the place of reciprocal unpaid relationships (Antaki, Finlay and Walton, 2008). The initial referral for psychotherapy nearly always comes through a third party, often a family member, a GP, a service manager or a member of a multi-disciplinary team, frequently without the person's knowledge. Psy-chotherapist Mark Haydon-Laurelut writes:

> ... the referral text is the site of relational discourses where the identity of the person with intellectual disabilities is fashioned, where narratives are created, power is exercised and the text's author and the person the text is about are positioned.
>
> (Haydon-Laurelut and Nunkoosing, 2010, p. 75)

He goes on to discuss such discourses that place adults with intellectual disabilities as being the site of problems and deficit, where their protests and resistance against such things as routinisation of daily life and institutional care practices are often interpreted as challenging behaviour that requires a therapeutic intervention to 'fix' (Haydon-Laurelut and Nunkoosing, 2010, p. 75). My initial experience of receiving such referrals brought my attention to the need to place respect for each person at the centre of the referral process – family, staff and client alike – where the power imbalance can be somewhat rectified. There is an even greater need to ensure respect within the therapeutic frame, where the client is often habituated to being powerless within professional care relationships. In my countertransference, Steven's intense stare at being offered choice regarding staying or leaving the therapy space activated feelings within me of deep uncertainty, fear and scepticism that we could possibly work together in relationship.

Steven did choose to attend his therapy sessions from then on, and for several years to come. That first session sparked his curiosity and also contained a level of humour that arose from my own lack of therapeutic experience at the time. I actually bargained with Steven that if he wanted to choose spitting as a means of communicating, that was fine with me, I would reciprocate with a water pistol. I produced the pistol and he looked at me in astonishment. He spat, I fired (thankfully both out of range of each other) and he guffawed. Thinking back on those moments, I wince a little at my own naiveté as I hadn't fully considered the depth of distress behind his action and how my response might be received as yet another murderous attack on the fragility of his being. However, my risk taking playfulness created an opportunity to redefine spitting as possibly having more meanings than a nonverbal communication of rage from a very hurt and desolate young man. In the following years, we developed an understanding within our shared communications that his warning pretend spit signified anger or frustration, often at my misunderstanding or misinterpretation. I learned to acknowledge, retreat (both metaphorically and physically) and apologise as I attempted to untangle the miscommunication in the cycle of rupture and repair upon which sense of self, trust in relationship and emotional resilience are built (Winnicott, 2002; Siegel, 2020). Sometimes my efforts were in vain and a spit would be sent in my direction, landing with careful aim at my feet, or perhaps on my leg if his anger at not being understood was too great, but this too disappeared over time as we co-created a language of nonverbal utterances and sounds for Steven's voice to be heard. The pretend spit took on a complexity of meanings linked with our facial expressions, the prosody of our vocalisations, and our embodied presence in that moment. This brings to mind psychiatrist and neurobiologist Stephen Porges' Polyvagal Theory (Porges, 2011) where he has traced the connection of the vagus nerve between the heart and the face,[3] and how attuned facial expression, prosody and vagally regulated therapeutic presence can activate the social engagement system rather than the fight, flight survival mechanisms of dorsal vagal activation (Porges, 2011, p. 125).

This development led to Steven's consented sharing of his meanings with his care team, providing a conduit to more attuned communication and understanding of his emotional life. It effectively reduced the transference of their potential anxiety, fear, disgust and rage when in his presence.

Working therapeutically with clients with an intellectual disability often necessarily requires the involvement of others, whether family members or members of their care team, to support their engagement in the psychotherapeutic process. As a result of many experiences where organisational pressures negatively impacted on the course of therapy, my current systemic model began to evolve through Alan Corbett's guidance, building on his integrated approach which he had developed as part of his work in forensic psychotherapy (Corbett 2014, p. 21). Fundamental elements became established, such as initiating inclusive, client directed conversation from the outset rather than the 'being spoken about' conversations that often take place between others in the client's presence; where seeking client consent and offering choice were embedded within support systems rather than being an afterthought, or a missing link. Concurrently, respectful support began to be offered to care staff and/or family members, with psycho-education and a reflective space as a pre-therapy requisite in order for them not only to understand the rationale behind the basic concepts such as client confidentiality, the right to privacy, and choice regarding attendance, but also to enhance relational connections rather than focusing on behavioural management. More importantly, it became evident that trauma informed care is necessary to fully support a person with an intellectual disability not only in therapy, but in their everyday lives.

Trauma

Over the years, it became apparent that ongoing staff training in trauma-informed care was a vital element in maintaining the safety and integrity of the client's therapy, along with making a significant positive impact on others' understanding of behaviours that were otherwise puzzling and sometimes frightening.

Anna was a young non-verbal woman with a severe intellectual disability who lived in a residential setting. She was referred to me because of increasingly aggressive behaviour linked to what appeared to be psychotic episodes. It was reported that in recent months she had limited all activity to walking incessantly in and out of rooms, up and down corridors, always seeking a staff member to link arms with in her nonstop walking. Inexplicably she would suddenly drag the person to the ground with an incredibly strong grip that was impossible to escape from without help. Anna would then sob inconsolably for hours. I visited her residential home, planning to arrange a series of assessment therapy sessions in order to build emotional attunement and ascertain Anna's capacity to consent to engage in therapy. At that first visit to introduce myself and the notion of therapy, I offered to be her walking companion. We began the circuit of the house; all external doors were locked because of what had been described as her obsessional need to escape. She first brought me to one such door, tried the handle and wanted to check my pockets, I presumed for a key. I explained I had no key, but I acknowledged her intense desire for the door to be opened and joined her in frustrated frowning at the lock with no key. We continued walking relatively slowly as I maintained what felt like a soliloquy while Anna's eyes darted everywhere with only occasional glances at my face. I felt a sudden pressure on my arm as she fiercely grasped me, so I followed the impulse of her movement without resistance and we both sank to the ground. I could feel her terror as she clung to me, so I used my voice to speak to her in the prosody of motherese (Malloch and Trevarthen, 2009) and softened my own muscle tone as she clung to me. She gradually relaxed her hold, and the sobbing started. We remained on the ground, with me instinctively shielding her body from the line of sight of the staff members who had come running. I reassured everyone all was fine, I needed no help and Anna and I would remain right here for a while, until Anna was ready to stand up again, which she did after several minutes. We resumed our walking until it was time for me to leave.

Our therapy sessions took place within the house because organisationally it was not possible to overcome the complexities of travelling to another destination with someone who was considered too volatile, uncooperative and a flight risk. After very intricate consideration of boundaries and containment within a mobile therapeutic frame, our therapy room became the intersubjective space between us as we continued walking together with occasional pauses in an empty room that had been made available to us. The next week, Anna modified her behaviour with me as her hyperaroused alarm response (Porges, 2011) no longer pulled us to the floor, but she drew me in front of her as she cowered in towards the wall. In a flash of realisation, I noticed that her terror was being triggered by another resident who had walked very quietly up behind us. I mentioned this to a staff member, who immediately recognised this as a kind of game he had noticed that the other resident played with Anna, creeping up and then touching her gently, making her jump. The staff member agreed that this was not an appropriate game to allow to happen to someone who was so obviously in a state of extreme hypervigilance and it ceased, but Anna's concerning behaviour didn't decrease.

Around this time, a quite horrific act was witnessed by a care worker passing by a window of the residential home. Another staff member was seen quietly approaching Anna from behind, wrestling her to the ground and then dragging her along the floor into her bedroom. The alarm was raised, a criminal investigation and conviction ensued. Anna was left with the sequelae of a trauma no-one had dared to imagine. It is beyond the scope of this chapter to delve any more deeply into the actions of the perpetrator, or to wonder about the enactment contained within the other resident's game. However, what has been replayed in so many situations is the existence of trauma where someone is referred because of perceived unacceptable behaviour, and is in fact desperately trying to wordlessly communicate his or her distress.

I was asked to assess Evan, a 12-year-old, who had begun to pull down his trousers and rub his naked bottom against a very loved teaching assistant's legs. Hormonal changes, approaching puberty and emerging sexual interest were all offered as explanations for this behaviour that horrified everyone and repelled his teaching assistant. In the transference, everyone was quite correct in identifying the strong sexualised message underneath his strange actions, but no-one had considered the possibility that Evan was trying to communicate through demonstration that something awful was happening in his life, and in fact a visiting uncle was sexually abusing him at home. The immediate leap to the defended position of a perception of the hypersexuality of the disabled (Liddiard, 2017), the alternative to the perception of asexuality previously mentioned, meant that the unbearable could remain unthought by those witnessing Evan's actions.

Research shows that internationally, children and adults with disabilities are three to four times more likely to be abused than the general population (Sullivan and Knutson, 2000; Stalker and McArthur, 2012). Numbers may be significantly higher as so many cases are unrecognised, minimised or simply not reported (Corbett, 2014). An Irish social work study (Flynn, 2020) identifies the attitudinal problems inherent in this: disabled teenagers are asexual and consequently will not be abused; disabled children's rights are replaced by sympathy; an over-empathy with parents' wishes and desires replaces action on behalf of the disabled child; higher thresholds tend to be required in order for action to be taken than for children without disabilities, and a general lack of recognition of the capacity for people to offend against someone with an intellectual disability. Despite having garda (Irish police) specialist interviewers available to them, day services and residential centres tend to carry out investigations 'in house', what Alan Corbett refers to as a siege mentality and consequently language is used to 'mislabel crimes as "inappropriate sexual behaviours" … and is a shocking denial of the traumatising impact of sexual abuse upon the victim' (Corbett, 2013). This knowledge deeply impacted on the direction my work began to take and I started to focus more on both teaching and clinical supervision, offering specialist support to other therapists, clinicians and agencies working in the area of trauma. This included succeeding Alan as a core trainer in the Garda specialist interviewing training, which he had been instrumental in setting up in 2007 and had asked me to continue, to ensure therapeutic thinking would underpin all learning in this vital work.

Trauma is an inherent part of disability psychotherapy, both the intrapsychic trauma of the disability itself (Sinason, 2010) and the interpsychic trauma of a world that often doesn't allow for an intersubjectivity based on respect and equality. A psychotherapy that is grounded in relationship, meeting the person at the developmental level appropriate to them in each moment of connection, of necessity cannot depend on spoken word alone. Neurobiological understandings of consciousness, the unconscious and growth of mind have given enormous value to creativity and play-based interactions in bringing about therapeutic change where trauma is present.

Intersubjectivity, the Unconscious and Creativity

Neuropsychologist and psychotherapist Allan Schore's research into affect regulation is particularly relevant to therapeutic work in the field of intellectual disability. He has shown that change mechanism is not necessarily mediated by insight, but is the product of an experience of therapeutic synchrony. He states that 'psychotherapy is not the "talking cure" but the affect communicating and regulating cure' (Schore, 2009, p. 128). In the transference and counter transference between client and therapist, affects are communicated through right brain emotional relational processes, not through language.

Schore goes on to explain that in order to know about the client's unconscious process, we need to pay attention to the embodied intersubjective dance that we both share, where breathing, muscle tone, hesitations, eye gaze and all outward expressions of our inward states lead to synchrony, or not. The ensuing pattern of engagement, arousal, withdrawal and re-engagement is the early pattern of attachment connection that underlies emotional regulation in relationship. This is especially important where there has been relational trauma:

> ... the sensitive empathic therapist allows the patient [sic] to re-experience dysregulating affects in affectively tolerable doses in the context of a safe environment, so that overwhelming traumatic feelings can be regulated and integrated into the patient's emotional life.
>
> (Schore, 2009, p. 130)

The inclusion of this intersubjectivity into scientific investigation has heralded a new era, and discoveries have been made that have revolutionised the scientific understanding of brain growth and development. Schore speaks of the 'paradigm shift from behaviour, to cognition, to bodily based emotion' (2012, p. 4) in which scientific research has transitioned from studies of language-based cognitive processes and voluntary motor functions, to emotional processing and embodied systems independent of cognitive processes. It makes it possible to move from the realm of the cognitive and analytical to the realm of experience-based emotional growth, where relationship is paramount.

This is of huge significance when looking at the importance of psychotherapy as an effective intervention not only for people with intellectual disabilities, but also for those without disabilities who have been deeply traumatised. Words are not enough. However, through a therapeutic intersubjectivity that is embodied and relational, a full spectrum of needs from the development of interpersonal relationships to the treatment of complex trauma can be successfully met. The role of play and creativity is a prime element in this, bringing about therapeutic change for both children and adults. Play therapy techniques are easily adaptable to match developmental levels throughout the lifespan, and creative arts, music, and movement are an intrinsic part of my clinical practice (McGrath, 2019). Schore states:

> Therapy focuses on interactively regulating conscious and unconscious negative and positive affect, as well as facilitating the growth of the patient's symbolic, imaginative functions. Play allows the patient and therapist not only to discover but to nurture different and more complex aspects of the right brain self.
>
> (Schore, 2019, p. 241)

Neurobiologically informed therapeutic practice that focuses on relationship not only provides an alternative evidence base to the reductionist notion of quantifiable change usually only contained in more cognitively based therapies, but also enriches our theoretical knowledge and provides a rationale for the inclusion of creativity that can often be misunderstood as only applicable within the realm of child psychotherapy.

Concluding Thoughts

Looking back has given me the opportunity to be thankful for those supervisors, psychotherapists and clinicians who have shaped and encouraged my clinical practice so far, and to deeply appreciate the relationships with all of my clients along the way. Their sharing of their inner worlds and their ability to survive and grow despite even the most adverse circumstances has humbled and awed me time and time again. My early days in getting to know and understand what life is actually like for someone with a disability has led me through academic, clinical and intersubjective discoveries that shape the way forward. The future holds hope, as the growing awareness of the need for trauma-informed care and for the provision of psychotherapy for people with disabilities is opening new avenues for teaching, consultation and clinical practice. As disability psychotherapy tends to focus on relationship at the deepest, most fundamental human level, without necessarily relying on words, it provides a rich ground for finding valuable ways to interpersonal connection in all psychotherapeutic encounters, regardless of ability.

Notes

1 Respond is the foremost organisation in the United Kingdom for the provision of psychotherapeutic services to people with disabilities who are affected by abuse, violence or trauma. See https://respond.org.uk/
2 Fiona Kumari Campbell (2009, p. 5) defines ableism as a network of beliefs, processes and practices that produces a particular kind of self and body, 'the corporeal standard' that is projected as perfect, species typical and therefore essential and fully human. It embodies a moral grammar that leaves disabled people at or beyond the very margins of society, refusing to recognise their value or esteem, their differences and competencies.
3 Porges' research has been invaluable in understanding the physiological underpinnings of both trauma and social engagement, and how this knowledge can be translated into a deeper awareness of emotional regulation and dysregulation in the therapy room. The heart face connection includes considering the muscles of the face (emotional expression), the eyelids (for social gaze and gesture), the middle ear muscles (for distinguishing the human voice from background sounds) and the laryngeal and pharyngeal muscles (for vocalising, swallowing, breathing).

Bibliography

Antaki, C., Finlay, W. M. L. and Walton, C. (2007). The staff are your friends: intellectually disabled identities in official discourse and interactional practice. *British Journal of Social Psychology, 46*: 1–18.
Alvarez, A. (1992). *Live Company. Psychoanalytic Psychotherapy with Autistic, Borderline, Deprived and Abused Children*. London: Routledge.
Alvarez, A. (2012). *The Thinking Heart. Three Levels of Psychoanalytic Therapy with Disturbed Children*. London: Routledge.
Bakhtin, M. (1984). *Rabelais and His World*. Indiana: Indiana University Press.
Campbell, F. K. (2009). *Contours of Ableism: The Production of Disability and Ableness*. London: Palgrave Macmillan.
Corbett, A. (2009). Words as a second language: the psychotherapeutic challenge of severeintellectual disability. In T. Cottis (ed.), Intellectual Disability, Trauma and Psychotherapy (pp. 45–62). London: Routledge.
Corbett, A. (2014). *Disabling Perversions. Forensic Psychotherapy with People with Intellectual Disabilities*. London: Karnac.
Corbett, A. (2016). *Psychotherapy with Male Survivors of Sexual Abuse*. London: Karnac.
Corbett, A. (ed.) (2019). *Intellectual Disability and Psychotherapy: The Theories, Practice and Influence of Valerie Sinason*. London: Routledge.

Corbett, A., Cottis, T. and Morris, S. (eds.) (1996). *Witnessing, Nurturing, Protesting. Therapeutic Responses to Sexual Abuse of People with Learning Disabilities.* London: David Fulton Publishers.

Cozolino, L. (2017). *The Neuroscience of Psychotherapy. Healing the Social Brain* 3rd edn. New York: Norton.

Flynn, S. (2020). Theorizing disability in child protection: applying critical disability studies to the elevated risk of abuse for disabled children. *Disability & Society*, 35(6), 949–971.

Foucault, M. (1991). *Discipline and Punish: The Birth of the Prison.* London: Penguin.

Garland-Thomson, R. (2009). *Staring: How We Look.* Oxford: Oxford University Press.

Goodley, D., Lawthom, R. and Runswick, C. K. (2014). Posthuman disability studies. *Subjectivity*, 7, 342–361.

Haydon-Laurelut, M. and Nunkoosing, K. (2010). I want to be listened to: systemic psychotherapy with a man with intellectual disabilities and his paid supporters. *Journal of Family Therapy*, 32, 73–86.

Hughes, B. (2012). Civilising modernity and the ontological invalidation of disabled people. In: D. Goodley, B. Hughes, and L. Davis (eds). Disability and Social Theory: New Developments and Directions (pp. 17–32). London: Palgrave Macmillan.

Liddiard, K. (2017). *The Intimate Lives of Disabled People.* London: Routledge.

Longmore, P. (2009). The second phase. From disability rights to disability culture. In R. Baird, S. Rosenbaum, S. Kay Tombs (eds.), Disability. The Social, Political and Ethical Debate (pp. 141–150). New York: Prometheus Books.

Malloch, S. and Trevarthen, C. (eds.). (2009). *Communicative Musicality: Exploring the Basis of Human Companionship.* Oxford: Oxford University Press.

McGrath, E. (2012). Dancing with Disability: An Intersubjective Approach. In D. Goodley, B. Hughes, and L. Davis. Disability and Social Theory. New Developments and Directions. New York: Palgrave Macmillan.

McGrath E. (2013). Beyond Integration. Reformulating Physical Disability in Dance. PhD, University of Bedfordshire.

McGrath, E. (2019). Creativity and the analytic condition. Creative arts approaches within a psychoanalytic frame. In A. Corbett (ed.), Intellectual Disability and Psychotherapy: The Theories, Practice and Influence of Valerie Sinason (pp. 21–33). London: Routledge.

Porges, S. (2011). *The Polyvagal Theory: Neurophysiological Foundations of Emotions, Attachment Communication and Self Regulation.* New York: Norton.

Schore, A. (2009). Right brain affect regulation: an essential mechanism of development, trauma, dissociation and psychotherapy. In D. Fosha, D. Siegel, and M. Solomon (eds.), The Healing Power of Emotion: Affective Neuroscience, Development and Clinical Practice (pp. 112–144). New York: Norton.

Schore, A. (2019). *The Development of the Unconscious Mind.* New York: Norton.

Siegel, D. (2020) *The Developing Mind* 3rd edn. New York: Guilford Press.

Sinason, V. (2002) Some reflections from twenty years of psychoanalytic work with children and adults with a learning disability. *Disability Studies Quarterly*, 22(3), 38–45.

Sinason, V. (2010). *Mental Handicap and the Human Condition* rev. *edn.* London: Free Association Books.

Sinason, V. (2020). *The Truth About Trauma and Dissociation*. London: Confer Books.

Snyder, S. and Mitchell, D. (2006). Afterword: Regulated Bodies. Disability Studies and the Controlling Professions. In D. Turner and K. Stagg (eds.), Disability and Deformity. Oxford: Routledge.

Stalker, K. and McArthur, K. (2012). Child abuse, child protection and disabled children: a review of recent research. *Child Abuse Review, 21(1)*, 24–40.

Sullivan, P. M., and Knutson, J. F. (2000). Maltreatment and disabilities: A population-based epidemiological study. *Child Abuse and Neglect, 24(10)*, 1257–1273.

Winnicott, D.W. (2002). *Winnicott on the Child*. Cambridge, MA: Perseus Books Group.

Chapter 8

Becoming a Disability Psychotherapist

Angelina Veiga

This chapter describes the experience of becoming a disability psychotherapist as developed through supervision with Dr Alan Corbett. Disability psychotherapy is concerned about thinking and working in a respectful way with people with intellectual disabilities. The disability psychotherapist is aware of culture in its multiple meanings and is cognisant of sameness and difference in both the patient and therapist. It is a profoundly relational encounter. Alan's influence in my evolvement as a disability psychotherapist is rooted in finding courage to face what can seem insurmountable, unthinkable and unspeakable. It involves keeping in mind that it is highly likely that patients with intellectual disabilities experience repetitive relational trauma in various degrees and in different facets of their lives and this evokes feelings of powerlessness and despair. This includes thinking about how people with intellectual disabilities are massively projected into by others in their lives and by society.

Being a disability psychotherapist shapes my engagement with the practice of psychoanalytic psychotherapy through bringing a particular kind of sensitivity to the impact of relational trauma and its devasting effects on marginalised people. It cultivates an awareness of the need to consider patients who may not initially be seen as a candidate for psychotherapy as someone who can indeed make use of the work. The work of a disability psychotherapist, due to the nature of working with trauma, can feel at times to be an overwhelming and bleak experience. Supervision spaces are pivotal to the success of this endeavour with the supervisory experience with Alan being a fundamental experience in the trajectory of becoming the therapist I now am. In this chapter I will describe my understanding of what disability psychotherapy is, and the experience of practising as one to address the question: *What does it mean to be a disability psychotherapist?* Clinical examples are used throughout the chapter to illustrate this; care has been taken to maintain the patients' confidentiality to disguise the work we were involved in.

What is disability psychotherapy?

Disability psychotherapy is an evidence-based treatment approach concerned with providing psychotherapeutic support for people with disabilities. While

DOI: 10.4324/9781003646242-11

psychotherapy has not traditionally been considered as a treatment approach for people with intellectual disabilities, the practice of disability psychotherapy advocates that individuals with intellectual disabilities have rich and mature internal lives despite any cognitive impairments, and that people with intellectual disabilities can make use of and benefit from psychotherapy treatment (Beail, 1995; Beail et al., 2005). The use of a psychoanalytic approach endeavours to explore the individual's inner world in order to make meaning of past and present experiences and how these shape one's internal experience. The hope of the work is to promote insight, integration and the management of unbearable thoughts and emotional states for the patient which can achieve gains in one's emotional intelligence. As disability psychotherapists we wonder if treatment perhaps also leads to a lessening of the intellectual disability itself, should we consider that a cognitive impairment can be impacted upon by unresolved traumatic experiences leading to secondary defences.

Disability psychotherapy is a pluralistic discipline that encompasses a wide range of modalities. The diversity of these approaches reflects the wide range of levels of disability and trauma that present in the consulting room. The intention of a pluralistic application is to offer opportunities for flexible approaches to clinical work to aid understanding. It is characteristic of the work that the clinical presentation is usually not straight-forward owing to the nature and complexity of the disability and corresponding trauma history. In addition, because of the way trauma and disability together affect the mind of the clinician, disability therapy work requires many minds to come together to promote thinking and understanding. A process of taking in, and the ensuing shaping of each other's work within one's mind is required for the therapist to meet the individual needs of the patient.

A key feature of disability psychotherapy is that the clinical work is not wholly delineated to working with just patients with intellectual disabilities but naturally extends to those in their network. Others, notably Sinason (1992), Cottis and O'Driscoll (2009), and Corbett (2009, 2016) have written on how an intellectual disability can be experienced as a trauma, and about the defences that are needed by individuals, systems and organisations to defend against these painful traumatic experiences. Thinking about how these defences are employed at the individual and systems level is a key component of working as a disability psychotherapist. We recognise that members of the network are often pivotal to the person being able to access their treatment and that members of the network hold the power for the treatment to proceed or not. The network is viewed as a patient, and we attempt to offer consultation and reflective spaces to the members of the network to help them think about their roles in supporting the patient. This includes thinking about what the experience of the person with the intellectual disability may be like. The approach of treating the system as a whole (the system as a patient) has much in common with the work of child and adolescent psychoanalytic psychotherapists who treat the family as a patient when treating their child patients. We share the view of working with the network as often being a necessary and an integral part of the therapeutic work.

Without adequate supervision and thinking spaces made available to key supports such as organisational staff members the treatment is under considerable threat of extinction. In addition, when there is no secure funding arrangement in place, which is unfortunately often the case, the treatment resides in a precarious position of danger of being annihilated. Supervision, consultation to the network and secure funding arrangements that include having opportunities to review with the network are helpful in sustaining the life of the treatment. Without these key supports being in place the therapy is in danger of being killed off, just as the person with an intellectual disability is killed off in society's mind. Often at these times of crisis in the life of the therapy the disability psychotherapist is thrust into role of advocate. As disability psychotherapists we acutely feel the pain and trauma of the loss, or potential loss of the treatment for our patients. Often we are in touch with the potent feelings of uncertainty and insecurity as these conflict with the sustainment of hope in the potentiality of the treatment to bring about psychic change for the patient.

The key tenets of working as a disability psychotherapist

Being a disability psychotherapist necessitates the ability to stay with the experience of being human in its many complexities, and to be in touch with aspects of this experience that are extremely painful and which we would prefer to disavow. Sinason (1992) has written eloquently on how people with intellectual disabilities are powerfully projected into, and what they may do to defend against what this evokes in them. As therapists we are not immune to enactments of projecting into our patients either. In his seminal book on forensic psychotherapy with people with intellectual disabilities Corbett (2014, p. 155) writes:

> forensic disability psychotherapy is an intersubjective process that involves the meeting of two minds and the creation of an intersubjective field in which differences can be tolerated, thought about, and made sense of. The key difference is that of ability – one mind is disabled and the other is not. The mutative power of the mind should allow the seemingly non-disabled mind to recognise its disabled parts and the disabled mind to become more open to thought and reflection.

By drawing attention to the need to tolerate, think about and metabolise experiences of difference the therapist and patient are able to create a shared understanding about their experiences together in the consulting room. The emphasis is on thinking together instead of enacting a paranoid schizoid defence to void one or both of the pain of the trauma of the disability. Crucially no one mind is privileged over the other. Rather it is the coming together of the two minds that promotes thinking about an abled and disabled experience. In this sphere both participants can learn something about themselves by means of the other during the clinical encounter. For the therapist this learning continues to be built upon in forums such as supervision, personal analysis and self-analysis. The experience of containment for the therapist promotes the thinking that is needed to be able to stay with the experience of disability. This supports the therapist to metabolise the clinical encounter without resorting to projecting into the patient as a defensive measure against being close to the experience of trauma and disability.

Sinason (1992) introduced many insightful concepts which help deepen our understanding of the psychological impact of intellectual disability. The 'handicapped smile' (p. 123) suggests that one has to smile and be compliant, but underneath the façade tremendous pain, loss and grief is lurking that needs to be defended from. In the first session with a young man with a moderate intellectual disability, as he sat down in his chair across from me he broke out into a huge smile. I wondered with him about the smile and he told me that he smiles all the time. He went on to say that he had not been smiling the day before because a peer from school followed him and his friend home and physically attacked them on the street. Despite his attempts he could not make it stop. It felt shocking and brutal. The patient immediately brought the experience of being oppressed, unseen and projected into in the first moment of us coming together, and how utilising the handicapped smile defended against these painful experiences. In my counter-transference in this first moment of meeting I already felt baffled, concerned and not sure what to do.

Another feature Sinason alerts us to is the employment of the primary disability as a 'secondary handicap' (p. 97). This occurs when the organic disability is exaggerated and used as a defence, and as a respite against living with the trauma of the disability. This can be seen where the individual behaves in a way where the organic disability appears to be much greater than it may actually be. With one patient with a moderate intellectual disability and autism we discovered that his inertia which greatly impacted on being able to do things like get out of bed in the morning resulted in him often missing out on activities he enjoyed such as going to a fitness class at his local gym. Over a long period of time we eventually moved from him feeling that it was 'because of my conditions' (meaning the intellectual disability and autism) to understanding it as a defensive mechanism against facing aspects of himself that are depressed and depleted and that need to be gathered up by someone else. In the counter-transference I often felt angry with him. My being in touch with this feeling of anger helped us think together about the self-destructive feelings he possessed that stopped things that could be helpful for him from occurring.

When a child with an intellectual disability is born it obscures the ordinary and important phantasy of the beautiful baby. The ability to mourn this may be severely compromised, if not impossible to do. Hate, shame and guilt for and about the intellectual disability can become entrenched in the family's psyche and subsequently projected into the person with the disability. Emanuel (1997, p. 281) writes:

> There is an absence of the phantasied beautiful baby, and instead of a thinking link being formed, and an ongoing effort being made to know and understand her baby (Bion's concept of 'K', 1962), reality is distorted, misrepresented or denied. The baby is not seen for who she actually is, and not only suffers from inadequate containment of projections but is often a receptacle for mother's projections of disappointment and loss.

As disability psychotherapists we are often working with the consequences of these projections and projective identifications that are present from birth or even before. For some then employing a secondary disability can become a means for psychic survival. Part of therapy work entails offering a containing experience for the patient so that these projections which are experienced as a trauma can be understood and worked through. When this is possible, alternative ways of thinking about oneself and being can be discovered and explored through the therapeutic relationship. This brings about a strengthening of ego development and a lessening of an identification of being disabled.

The disability therapy framework

Generally people enter into psychotherapy treatment when they are in a state of crisis. This is no different for people with intellectual disabilities, although they are seldom the ones to initiate the treatment. An important difference in the practice of disability psychotherapy is that treatment tends to be inaugurated by someone in the network who holds a concern for the individual, often a parent or agency. Treatment is often instigated by others to help manage self injurious behaviour, grief, loss and mourning, experiences of sexual abuse or the risk of it, or engagement in sexualised or seriously harmful behaviours, amongst other concerns. Disability psychotherapy recognises that risky or harmful behaviours are a symptom and communication of psychological distress, and while a reduction in these behaviours is ideal they are not the focus of the therapy. Instead the focus of the therapy is to support unmanageable thoughts and feelings to become tolerable, thus facilitating personal growth and self-understanding, and an easing of the intellectual disability being used in a defensive way. Concurrently a reduction or cessation of risky or harmful behaviours may come about as new ways of being emerge.

As people with intellectual disabilities are usually brought to treatment instead of seeking it out themselves, disability psychotherapists assess consent for treatment with the patient in a similar way that one does with child patients. Usually this is done over a series of assessment sessions so that explicit consent over implied consent can be evidenced as part of a relational experience. Consent may also be revisited at times when confidentiality may need to be widened out such as when risk and safeguarding concerns arise, or at times of review such as with members of the network or as part of the funding arrangement when progress reports are required by the funders. These intrusions in the clinical space may evoke anxieties from both the patient and therapist about the robustness of treatment and bring threats of annihilation of it. At these times careful thinking needs to occur in therapy sessions and in supervision in order to safeguard the therapeutic relationship and the clinical work. The voice of the patient is paramount in thinking about how to manage the intrusion into the frame. The therapist may have to communicate strongly to the network how serious and significant these intrusions are and how damaging they can be.

Disability psychotherapy usually occurs through the use of regularly scheduled psychotherapy sessions. We offer the same setting, both internal and external, to our patients with disabilities as we do to our patients without disabilities, although we may modify the setting to support creative ways of working if necessary. The patients I saw for treatment as I was evolving into a disability psychotherapist under Alan's guidance were seen in the private consulting rooms I shared in a mainstream psychotherapy practice in a city centre location. My patients were treated in a private, community setting just like anyone else I might see. This was vital as it promoted the acceptance and integration of people with intellectual disabilities as having the opportunity to access ordinary psychotherapy treatment just like anyone else. It also challenged the practice of people with intellectual disabilities only being seen in specialist services, as if they should remain hidden away from society. With the external setting established it is then possible to work the way we normally would albeit with some modifications, such as the use of art materials or toys.

Our internal setting is monitored through supervision, self-analysis and our discussions with likeminded colleagues. Our therapeutic aim remains to carefully observe, recognise and interpret the individual's thoughts, feelings, dreams, nightmares, fantasies, anxieties, behaviours and any non-verbal communications just as we would with any other patient. Crucially it is not a prerequisite for the therapy for the patient to have verbal communication. Disability psychotherapists are skilled at using different methods to communicate with and understand their patients.

A pivotal ability the disability psychotherapist hones is developing sensitivity to one's own counter-transference, and to the disability transference. Disability transference is a phenomenon where the therapist's capacity to process is affected: namely the therapist just cannot think, feels stupefied and confused and is unable to act with agency (Corbett, 2009; 2014). Working with disability transference requires the exploration of the clinician's counter-transference responses which in turn assist in uncovering the unconscious communications and projective processes at play within the clinical situation. Some of the manifestations of the disability transference include sleepiness, failure to retain thought, temptation to act rather than think, breaking time boundaries, boredom, somatic responses, a desire to deny disability, confusion and a disabled dissociation (Corbett, 2014, pp. 84–85). A sensitive awareness to one's own counter-transference facilitates the therapist to intuitively access the projected and projective identification aspects of the therapeutic encounter so that they can be contained, thought about and made sense of with the patient, and in supervision. With one patient with a moderate learning disability I felt, almost immediately on the patient's arrival, his vulnerability about the time we would spend away from each other during the upcoming holiday period. I was also confronted by something erotic in his physical presentation that I could not seem to understand. In supervision Alan and I thought it was likely that on the verge of a separation, the initial referrer's reasons may come to my mind serving as a reminder of the patient's vulnerability and potency to act out during a separation. This experience of feeling abandoned during time away from therapy is extremely painful for this patient. It likely unconsciously mirrors earlier infantile experiences of being abandoned. In the counter-transference, through a projective identificatory experience, I was in touch with his vulnerability. This created a worry in me about what could happen in the upcoming gap in the therapy which I needed help to understand, enabling it to be thought about and contained for the patient.

Identifying as a disability psychotherapist

Many psychotherapists are working psychotherapeutically with people with intellectual disabilities. However, it is important politically to conceptualise and call myself a disability psychotherapist. Identifying as a disability psychotherapist promotes the work of disability psychotherapy as something in addition to working as a psychotherapist. It requires an overt commitment to this patient group, and importantly to the understanding to the particular needs of patients with intellectual disabilities. Interestingly, being a disability psychotherapist is not separate to who I am as an adult psychotherapist or a child and adolescent psychoanalytic psychotherapist. It does not manifest differently in how I work as a clinician. Instead, the identification of being a disability psychotherapist retains a particular place in my mind when I think about my work. When people ask me about my work I include how I also work with people with intellectual disabilities. This promotes the work of therapy with this patient group, and it acknowledges that being a disability psychotherapist is a fundamental component of my professional identity. Indeed when I initially trained as an adult psychotherapist my first training case was with a woman with intellectual disabilities and autism who was experiencing loss. This experience of working with intellectual disability and autism in my first training profoundly shaped my clinical interests and the direction of my therapeutic endeavours since.

Like other authors in this book I do not, to my knowledge, have a link to intellectual disability that I am consciously aware of. However, it has always been important to me to work with marginalised people who have been affected by trauma. I suspect this links to the experience of migration within my own family history. In my work I naturally find myself taking up the position of an advocate. It warrants that I have to be mindful of the pull to and also the need for the role of an advocate. Corbett (2014) warns of the split emotional reaction to working with the trauma of disability. In some cases therapists can be lured into excessive involvement in helping the patient. Conversely there can be an avoidance of and distancing from the problem personified and carried by the patient. The disability psychotherapist also has to consider what potentially may be enacted by all involved in the endeavour of disability psychotherapy. When there are anxieties within the network, for example, when a network worries that something sexually harmful may occur should the patient even express a sexual fantasy, this can impede on the person accessing treatment or being supported to continue with treatment. The therapist may then have to strongly advocate for treatment as something extremely beneficial in understanding the psychic life of the patient, and work vigorously to contain the anxieties of the network such as by offering formal or informal reflective thinking spaces.

Alan's influence on my development as a disability psychotherapist

Alan was a generous and humble colleague and teacher. He was astute, kind and encouraging. I was fortunate to meet him shortly after my adult psychotherapy training ended when I was working in Dublin and was in need of a supervisor who understood what it was like to work as a disability psychotherapist, even though at the time I did not know yet that I was one. As a supervisee I had the benefit of Alan's unique focus on utilising a trauma-informed psychoanalytic approach as part of a core skill set as part of my development as a disability psychotherapist. This approach has assisted me to view my patients from a less pathologising stance, and to be more open and able to receive communications which can feel difficult, confusing or bizarre. With Alan's aid I began to work in a relational psychoanalytic way in order to consider the therapeutic encounter as a pivotal arena for psychic growth and healing. This remains a cornerstone of how I practice. Casement (1985) describes the phenomenon of the internal supervisor, and how over time one's supervisor may become an internalised helpful object who is integrated within one's own experience of being a psychotherapist. It is possible then to consult this internal supervisor in oneself during the live clinical encounter. Through supervision with Alan, I have embodied something of the quality of being with him, and this supports me to feel I can stay close to my patient's experiences and take relational risks.

Alan gave space, energy and focus to the *Secrets of Disability*. These *secrets* were developed independently, and concurrently by Sinason and Hollins who were finding out similar things at similar times. They were being enriched by each other and learning from one another. (Sinason, 2024). They came together to join together their ideas which cumulated in the five *Secrets of Disability* (Hollins and Sinason, 2000). As Alan's supervisee I had the benefit of his own unique focus on the *Three Secrets of Disability:* Disability, Sexuality, and Death (Hollins and Grimer, 1988). He reshaped and developed the original ideas he was learning about through collaboration with colleagues in the Institute of Psychotherapy and Disability (IPD) in order to make them in a way his own. He placed emphasis on the experience of dependency bound up within the disability and its impact on attachment and separation operating through projective identifications; societal disavowal of sexuality for people with intellectual disabilities and the unconscious belief of damage that is bound up within expressions of sexuality; and societal projection of death into people with intellectual disabilities as a mechanism of defending against difference and fear of the disabled parts within one's self.

Alan graciously shared his thinking with me as it applied to the clinical work we were discussing, making it a meaningful and powerful supervision encounter that was grounded in a community of likeminded colleagues. He encouraged the talking about the ideas we were discussing in supervision such as the *Three Secrets of Disability* in non-clinical settings. The aim was to widen out views on the experience of intellectual disability for professionals working within the field of disability. He advocated for a challenge of societal notions of intellectual disability in order to promote an unwavering belief, evidenced in his clinical work and others such as colleagues in the IPD that people with intellectual disabilities have rich internal worlds that need help to be understood just like any other patient. Therefore they too have a right to access psychotherapy treatment. In my clinical work I was finding evidence of this too enabling us to have rich and impassioned discussions.

Alan understood that from the beginning of a treatment there might be the possibility that the patient can hear a symbolic interpretation. Symbolic interpretations are indirect and figurative representations of the unconscious with interpretations being 'the verbal communication by the analyst of the hypothesis of an unconscious conflict that seems to have dominantly emerged now in the patient's communication in the therapeutic encounter' (Kernberg, 2016, p. 287). One patient with a moderate intellectual disability described in the first session the mess he had made with his sibling and how he had tidied it up. At the time I could not understand his communication and it left me feeling disabled. In supervision we thought about how my counter-transference may have been correct but was not understood yet. We wondered whether the patient may have been wondering whether he could bring a mess to his therapy, and whether I could tolerate it. Through Alan's teachings I learned how to gauge the fluidity of the disability – that is who feels able and who feels disabled – and how this moves between patient and therapist as a marker of fluctuating states of mind. This is an important form of projective identification that needs to be monitored closely to inform the work.

Living ghosts inside our minds

At that time of my immigration and therefore the ending of the supervision experience, Alan and I spoke about how when a therapy ends it can be as though the patients become living ghosts within our minds. He encouraged me to write about these experiences as I felt haunted particularly by a young man with an intellectually disability that I saw for a long treatment. Sometimes I thought I saw the patient on a London street. At these times it felt as though this patient was everywhere and sometimes even now I find myself thinking about him from time to time and wondering how he is. Later on when I trained as a child psychotherapist the idea of our patients becoming living ghosts in our minds became even more solidified for me as an organic, but nonetheless important and sometimes painful part involving the ending of the work.

When considering ghosts inside our minds it is important to think of these figures as not just haunting presences but also as friendly, supportive and helpful. When I began to write this chapter I felt at an impasse. I experienced Alan's death as a tremendous loss and I needed much help to move through my grief so that I could be in contact with the powerful and dynamic supervisory experience that was alive in me. Alan observed that with disability, and thus often in disabled organisations where the prevalence of disability can be considered a trauma, the systemic functioning is affected resulting in a paralysis of thought as a defence against the deliberating and often painful experience of having a disability (Corbett, 2011–2012). Valerie and I understood that the IPD had with Alan's death experienced a trauma and as a result this book in its own way developed a disability. Alan's death and other life and world events got into many of us in a way that made it difficult to think and progress with the project, and there was a need for much nurturing, mourning and metabolising to occur in order for this project to complete.

Through the working through of experiences of trauma and loss, growth and development emerged and flourished. In the IPD we all bear the burden of societal exclusion and the lack of adequate access for treatment for those with a disability. Because of this we care even more about our relationships with colleagues and our mutual support and understanding. The loss of a fine and irreplaceable colleague is felt by all of us but just as we work through the loss our patients face to feel the richness of potential so too can we enjoy the living legacy of Dr Alan Corbett.

Bibliography

Beail, N. (1995). Outcome of psychoanalysis, psychoanalytic and psychodynamic psychotherapy with people with intellectual disabilities: a review. *Changes*, 13, 186–191.

Beail, N., Warden, S., Morsley, K. and Newman, D. (2005). Naturalistic evaluation of the effectiveness of psychodynamic psychotherapy with adults with intellectual disabilities. *Journal of Applied Research in Intellectual Disabilities*, 18, 245–251.

Bion, W.R. (1962). *Learning from Experience*. London: Heinemann (reprinted London: Karnac, 1984).

Casement, P. (1985). *Learning from the Patient*. London: Routledge.

Corbett, A. (2009). Words as a second language: The psychotherapeutic challenge of severe intellectual disability. In Cottis, T. (Ed.), *Intellectual Disability, Trauma and Psychotherapy* (p.55). London: Routledge.

Corbett, A. 2011–2012. Personal Communication.

Corbett, A. (2014). *Disabling Perversions: Forensic Psychotherapy with People with Intellectual Disabilities*. Forensic psychotherapy monograph series. London: Karnac.

Corbett, A. (Ed.) (2019). *Intellectual Disability and Psychotherapy. The Theories, Practice and Influence of Valerie Sinason*. London: Karnac.

Cottis, T. (Ed.) (2009). *Intellectual Disability, Trauma and Psychotherapy*. London: Routledge.

Cottis, T. and O'Driscoll, D. (2009). Outside in: The effects of trauma on organisations. In Cottis, T. (Ed.), *Intellectual Disability, Trauma and Psychotherapy* (pp.82–83). London: Routledge.

Emanuel, L. (1997). Facing the damage together. *Journal of Child Psychotherapy*, 23 (2), 279–302.

Hollins, S. & Grimer, M. (1988). *Going Somewhere: People with Mental Handicap and Their Pastoral Care*. London: SPCK (Society for Promoting Christian Knowledge).

Hollins, S. & Sinason, V. (2000). Psychotherapy, learning disabilities and trauma: new perspectives. *British Journal of Psychiatry*, 176, 32–36.

Kernberg, O. (2016). The four basic components of psychoanalytic technique and derived psychoanalytic psychotherapies. *World Psychiatry*, 15(3): 287–288.

Sinason, V. (2024). Personal Communication.

Sinason, V. (1992). *Mental Handicap and the Human Condition: New Approaches from the Tavistock*. London: Free Association Books.

Section C

Applications of Disability Psychotherapy

Chapter 9

Understanding the Effects of Trauma in People with Intellectual Disability

Looking at Diagnosis of Post Traumatic Stress Disorder

Georgina Parkes

It is reported that people with an intellectual disability (ID) are at an increased risk of trauma, both in childhood and throughout their life. Sullivan and Knutson (2000) looked at over 50,000 school aged children and found those with a disability, particularly ID, were at the highest risk of abuse, and especially sexual abuse. Whether they are at increased risk of developing post-traumatic stress disorder (PTSD), complex PTSD and/or dissociative symptoms after experiencing trauma(s) is not so clearly reported, however there are indications that would suggest people with ID are at higher risk of developing these disorders.

The new diagnosis of complex PTSD in ICD (11) was formulated to be able to separate out those who will benefit from different types of treatments and therapies. For a review of the diagnoses of PTSD and complex PTSD in ICD (11) see Cloitre (2020). More people with ID are likely to experience recurrent trauma and adverse life events in their lifetime compared to the general population. Therefore, it could be argued, they are also more likely to have complex post-traumatic stress disorder and other sequelae. However, in my experience relatively few people with ID receive this diagnosis. I postulate here that this is often because traumas are not disclosed either by the person themselves or those around them. The symptoms may not fall into the traditional pattern of core PTSD. Furthermore, often there are several psychiatric diagnoses and physical health issues present, all of which seem more pressing or more likely to explain the difficulties. These include challenging behaviour, autism, ADHD, epilepsy, bipolar, traumatic head injury, psychotic episodes and so on. Hence trauma and PTSD are often missed. I argue here, however, that is it crucial to see the impact of trauma and make these diagnoses to guide towards treatment options. In this chapter, I will outline the reasoning behind these statements with some evidence and clinical examples which have been anonymised and demographic details changed to protect identities.

The lifetime prevalence of PTSD in the general population is 7%, with 80% of the population exposed to at least one traumatic event during their lifetime (De Vries and Olff, 2009; Kessler et al., 2005).

DOI: 10.4324/9781003646242-13

Seven percent of those people exposed to a traumatic event will develop PTSD in the general population, therefore you would expect similar levels or higher in the ID population given the increased rate of factors associated with developing PTSD and CPTSD.

In a meta-analysis of the prevalence of PTSD in ID, five studies were found and the pooled prevalence was 10%, which is at the upper limit of that seen in the general population (Daveney et al., 2019). It was recognised that whilst PTSD can be diagnosed it often goes unrecognised in people with ID.

We know that mental health problems in ID have been reported as two to four times higher and up to 75% higher than in the general population (Deb, Thomas and Bright, 2001; Moss and Patel, 1993; Buckles, Luckasson and Keefe, 2013). Parkes et al. (2007), found that of 100 patients' consecutive referrals for psychodynamic psychotherapy at the Joan Bicknell Centre, St George's Hospital, 27 were referred for trauma or abuse, 21 for challenging behaviour, and seven for sex offending behaviour. There was discussion that more people disclosed abuse during therapy who weren't referred for that reason, although this was a high rate as a referral reason (27% in a clinical population).

There is some evidence for lower developmental/intellectual level leading to higher risk of PTSD and more serious symptomatology (Macklin et al., 1998; McNally et al., 1995; Mevissen-Renckens and de Jongh, 2010). Also, a higher risk of sexual abuse is reported in a literature review of the ID population than in the general population (Byrne, 2018). Some studies show 6–20% higher rates than in the general population. It could be assumed that this would lead to higher levels of PTSD in traumatised individuals with ID than in the general population, but this appears not to be the case. Rather than accepting this I believe it is underdiagnosed in people with ID who present to services. Clinicians need to consider the option of trauma being present and be aware that it may not be volunteered; time and a trusting relationship may be needed before it can be discussed.

Adverse childhood experiences (ACE) studies show us how these experiences have a cumulative as well as a direct effect on risk behaviours and health problems (Felitti et al., 1998). These experiences can affect our physical health, auto immune problems, and anything from COPD and heart problems to substance misuse and mental illness. As the number of ACEs increases, the risk of every outcome in the domains of mental illness, substance abuse, sexual and aggressive offending increase, and the mean number of co-morbid outcomes triples across the range of the ACE score. This was a statistically significant result (Hughes et al., 2017).

Brain imaging studies using MRI show physiological effects of trauma on the brain (Lanius et al., 2010) such that trauma effects have become fixed in the mind. If you like, in a neurobiological rendering of Freud's trauma (Breuer and Freud, 1893), it is described as a psychical event that has left an unmetabolizable residue. Freud saw trauma as something that came from the outside, the memory of which lodged in the mind like a foreign object.

"Unprocessed fear" is a useful psychological descriptive term that aids us in understanding trauma but the nature of this unprocessed fear is very complex in its effects. Therapies for PTSD focus on processing fear and the traumatic events are more helpful with "core PTSD" for single traumatic events, on the background of no previous trauma rather than in complex PTSD (Matheson, 2016).

Powerlessness in early trauma can lead to overwhelming shame and self-blame which is highly resistant to change. Neuroscience also demonstrates the less common response to trauma of dissociation, numbness, freezing and depersonalisation (Lanius et al., 2010). People with ID who are less able to express themselves—whether they are non-verbal, have reduced language or have autism, or can be dependent, possibly, on their abuser—would be at increased risk as there is more likely to be a power imbalance.

Difficulties diagnosing PTSD in people with ID

In one study (Mason-Roberts et al., 2018) of PTSD in people with ID, 33 people were recruited who had full capacity to consent to the study, all of whom had a history of a traumatic event. So it is possible to make a diagnosis, however, this is just in higher functioning people with ID and also those where a history of one-off traumatic event was catastrophic, public or known about. However, it is not this group of people that I am discussing here. It is more those who are complex, who don't recover or get better when their mental illness or physical illness is treated, who maybe have epilepsy and non-epileptic/dissociative seizures. Those who, maybe, teams feel overwhelmed or exhausted by, with high levels of emotion, or cut off from, with a total lack of emotion. One criterion which must be present to diagnose PTSD is a history of traumatic event(s). In my experience, people with ID don't usually present to services by telling us of this or these events. For some people it is their normal living experience, or their past, something they see as unconnected to how they are now and not something to report or relate to the difficulties they are experiencing. There may be a long time delay from when the event or events occurred and when they are brought to, or come to the clinic seeking help. People can also feel too ashamed to speak. Whatever the reason, it is a major ethical dilemma that people are not getting diagnosed and therefore not getting the help they need. As a result, we need research into this area. Also, we need informed clinicians who keep this in mind. From personal experience and from researching this chapter, aggressive behaviour appears to be the most common symptom which is linked to trauma (McNally, Taggart and Shevlin, 2021). Hopefully the newer diagnostic category of complex PTSD will be a more helpful way of looking at the outcomes of repeated traumas and how they present in people with ID.

If we look through the psychiatric lens at PTSD in people with ID, McCarthy (2001) suggests that aggression, anger, sleeping problems, depression, self-harm and distractibility are presenting symptoms. Others suggest sexually inappropriate behaviours (Sobsey and Mansell, 1994; Mansell, Sobsey and Calder, 1992) social isolation, a poor sense of personal safety and low self-esteem (Mansell, Sobsey and Moskal, 1998). Additionally, there are many papers and books where people evidence their clinical experience but it is not evidenced in a formal study. In my experience a common occurrence seen as a presenting factor but not seen as diagnostic or related is repeated allegations which turn out to be unsubstantiated. It seems to be coming from an extreme dissociation and at the same time a trigger occurring which pushes them into almost a flashback situation which is experienced as really happening or at least a heightened fear of it really happening again, which is difficult to process and understand for the individual. There can also be a behaviour of repeatedly calling emergency services which can be linked to past trauma in those with ID.

Complex PTSD includes the same symptoms as PTSD and also three disturbances of self-organisation: emotional dysregulation, interpersonal difficulties and negative self-concept.

These can be seen as difficulty controlling emotions; being angry or distrustful; feeling emptiness or hopelessness, permanently damaged or worthless, or completely different to others; feeling that nobody can understand; avoiding friendships and relationships; and having dissociative symptoms, physical symptoms and suicidal feelings.

However, it is not discussed that when people come for help, they might find it difficult to link the traumatic events with their current behaviours. They—and this is particularly true for those with ID—do not put two and two together and therefore often neither they themselves or carers will volunteer information about a traumatic event in the past.

Issues in ID leading to higher risk of sequelae post-trauma

Prolonged exposure to trauma affects concept of self (Herman, 1992). This is already impaired in people with ID who typically develop this concept later. They may have to negotiate separating from care-givers and they may continue to be dependent on family or carers throughout their lives, which can affect how they see themselves as an individual.

Sexual abuse in childhood is much more likely to produce CPTSD (Karatzias et al., 2017a, 2017b). As we know people with ID are more likely to suffer sexual abuse.

Autism/ADHD

There are higher rates of ASD the lower the IQ. People with autism may experience traumatic reactions to events that might not be seen as traumatic to people who don't have autism (Brewin, Rumball and Happa, 2019), such as change in routine, social situations or sensory stimuli. It can be hard to work out what the issue is. For example, a high-pitched noise or leaf blower. Whatever it is, needs to be teased out so that things can be offered like ear defenders in this example. There can be problems in accessing treatment due to finding it hard to explain feelings and communicate their experiences which might be minimised or not taken seriously (Rumball, 2019). People with ADHD similarly experience sensory processing difficulties and also emotional dysregulation which those around them find difficult to manage and hence can become isolated and find it difficult to make friends. Often they are rejected by groups of children at school within minutes of meeting them (Barkley, Murphy and Fischer, 2008).

What is known about people with ID and the effects of trauma?

Thirty-three adults with mild to moderate ID were recruited from Community Learning Disability Teams in the UK (Mason-Roberts et al., 2018). They had to be able to give consent to the study and have a history of at least one traumatic life event. Of those in the study, 75% were taking psychotropic medication and 57% had a co-morbid condition. The mean number of life events was 4.55. No one had experienced just childhood life events, but some had experienced just adulthood events. Multiple traumatisation in people with ID was associated with an increased risk of depression and self-harm but not with increased risk of PTSD (core symptoms). In terms of being able to give consent, this would exclude some people with mild ID and moderate ID, and possibly all with severe ID. It is however a very important piece of research and shows the sheer amount of trauma suffered by people with ID and by reference how overwhelming it can be for professionals working in this field to accept this level of trauma. It does not surprise me that people did not meet criteria for PTSD as in ICD (10) and again I think this points to us needing different criteria to diagnose PTSD in people with ID.

Mevissen-Renckens and de Jong (2010) reviewed the literature on PTSD and ID. They found 18 papers in all and divided them into assessment, prevalence and treatment of PTSD in people with ID. Prevalence was extremely low and presentation was more like that seen in children with behavioural equivalents of symptoms such as self-harming behaviour. Information on the traumatic events of the past is often missing or unknown by current care givers. Lack of a validated assessment instrument in people with ID was also discussed. Four papers discussed in the literature review (Mevissen-Renckens and de Jong, 2010) had prevalence rates of PTSD (in a total of 359 people with ID) ranging from 2.5% to 60%. Large scale study information was lacking. However, these papers did show a link between trauma and PTSD in ID. Some support was found for the idea that people with ID are more vulnerable to developing PTSD and have more exposure to life events than in the general population. Treatment options discussed high rates of physical illness and mental health issues. Discussion was also around teaching to avoid triggers, creating a safe environment and the need for psychotherapy. Papers were found that used EMDR, CBT and psychodynamic therapy, all of which showed some positive outcomes (although these were mainly case reports).

The Lancaster and Northgate Trauma Scales (LANTS) for people with mild to moderate intellectual disability (Wigham, Hatton and Taylor, 2011) has been developed to try and measure effects of trauma in ID. This scale was used in a case study of five adults with moderate to severe intellectual disability in Norway (Bakken et al., 2014) which shows that PTSD diagnosis is possible using third party information, case notes and interviews using LANTS.

There is particularly scarce information about people with more severe disabilities.

The impact of events scale (IES) (Hall, Jobson and Langdon, 2014) has developed an intellectual disability version—the IES-ID, which is a self-report scale in which individuals are asked to firstly name an event then go through the questionnaire based on that event. As discussed before, this is problematic when the initial event(s) or later incident(s) may not be connected by the individual as a reason for their difficulties or may not be volunteered, in part possibly due to shame or stigma. Another reason is that carers do not volunteer the traumatic event as an issue.

Turk, Robins and Woodhead (2005) showed it was possible to diagnose and treat PTSD in two people with severe ID. Both had Fragile X syndrome and had suffered (separately) a road traffic accident; additionally one had autistic features and the other ADHD. However, I am not sure that it shows the core features of PTSD as claimed, but rather how difficult it is to diagnose PTSD without these. For both people it took some time for clinicians to work out they were suffering with PTSD and both suffered extreme distress which impacted on their quality of life and their family and carers. They used the pre-trauma functioning as a base line to make the diagnosis. This suggests that the core features of PTSD may rely, to some extent, on higher cognitive functioning and more sophisticated communication skills, such that people with more severe ID may not manifest these symptoms. Rather baseline functioning, history of a traumatic event prior to the change in baseline, subsequent alteration of emotional state or challenging behaviour would be enough to consider the diagnosis and instigate therapy. This centred on exposure therapy and work on locus of control and relaxation and was reported to be very successful in these two cases. As we have said before history of the event can be lacking but pre- and post-baseline functioning are important and when there is a change in behaviour then often a history of traumatic event can be teased out. For example, in one person I had to work quite hard over several visits to tease out a history of falling between a toilet and a radiator and suffering burns. The physical aspects were treated but as this event had occurred over a year previously, it had not been linked by carers to the current distress and depression which the person with severe ID was suffering from and which had gradually worsened over time. Diagnostic overshadowing and chronicity were both an issue in this case with caregivers not linking the traumatic event to the presentation.

Probability of more CPTSD in people with ID

As previously discussed, more people with ID than the general population have experienced sexual abuse and repeated trauma, with one study indicating a mean of 4.55 traumatic events. Repeated trauma increases the risk of complex PTSD rather than core PTSD which is more common after one traumatic event.

Some people with ID may already have had a life-threatening illness or a period of hospitalisation with a near death experience, e.g. cord around the neck at birth, being hit over the head with a hammer by a parent which caused their ID aged seven, falling down the stairs age three which caused their learning disability, heart problems in down syndrome, recurrent operations for a cerebral shunt. All these are a few examples from previous patients I have seen. They are more likely to have co-morbid physical health problems, risk of choking or indeed have choked. Indeed, ID in itself can be a traumatic event within a family (Hollins and Sinason, 2000) and psychologically for the person themselves in that they grow up to internalise negative views of themselves (Sinason, 2002; McNally, Taggart and Shevlin, 2021).

Ryan (1994) looked at 310 consecutive people with developmental disability (a North American term which approximately corresponds with ID in UK) seen in a clinic for complicated behaviours. Of these, 51 were subsequently diagnosed with PTSD. The paper described usually at least two types of abuse in each person with PTSD. Most sexual abuse happened over a prolonged period by multiple perpetrators in childhood. Of these cases, 66% were women and the average age was 33. Half were non-verbal and almost all were referred for violent behaviour.

Most commonly there was no previous psychiatric diagnosis other than the behaviour or schizophrenia in some cases. Less common was autism and a range of other prior diagnoses. In half of these at least one traumatic event was known to someone working with the client but was not volunteered to the professional. 66% had a medical illness. Some people with developmental disability communicated through drawings, gesture or someone who knew them well as a communication partner, whereas some could report through verbal means solely.

Treatment centred on six areas and all 23 who had access to all six areas showed improvement.

Firstly was use of medication to treat co-morbid mental illness. Secondly was treatment of physical health problems. Barriers for treatment were discussed with physicians often reluctant to provide input due to the ID. The third aspect of treatment was looking at side effects of medications already prescribed and over prescription and reducing these. Fourth was psychotherapy, which was often initially denied due to the person's disability and an idea that people with ID "forget trauma". This also involved assisting people with ID with how to stay safe.

Fifth was an attempt to control dissociative triggers, by monitoring the environment for olfactory, visual, tactile or auditory triggers or making changes of environment to reduce them. Discussion around safety was also undertaken; horrifyingly, some people were still encouraged to have unsupervised contact with their abusers. Certainly, this has been my experience when staff don't know the history at all. In one patient, their father was dying and there was a big effort by carers to take the patient to visit him in a care home. There was no indication of knowledge of the horrific childhood abuse suffered by this patient at the hands of the father. Instead, there was a pressure to visit. Indeed, in my experience it is often services who forget the trauma, not the person with the ID.

Whilst we may not always be able to monitor the environment for triggers well, the concept of a safe base that is needed prior to therapy would be a useful way of providing this. Sometimes people need to move for this to be provided.

Finally was education and support for staff, education in PTSD, and support and emergency backup systems for out of hours care. Staff also need to feel safe and supported.

This approach, peeling back the layers of the onion, is a helpful model of treatment for complex cases with presumed and known trauma and challenging behaviour. I did, however, experience tertiary trauma from reading the case examples in this paper, waking up at 5am thinking of them. It is important to know that hearing either first hand or as a supervisor or even reading about trauma can cause effects in the listener, and we all need support, to feel held and have safe spaces to continue the work. It is also important to acknowledge our experiences and seek independent help when needed. This is so that we don't either act it out unconsciously, or feel we have no alternative but to leave the work to others. Whilst I don't want to get into a discussion here I do want to say that these dynamics can be at the heart of scandals in institutional care. Perhaps it is a topic for a future chapter.

Team and family dynamics

Sometimes, there can be a dynamic within the team of professionals saying a traumatised patient has nothing really wrong with them and can be discharged. People are often acting from a lack of feeling projected into them by the patient who is trying to dissociate from the trauma. Sometimes of course it is from a secondary traumatisation that the professional is experiencing and reacting against unconsciously, because it is hard to be in touch with trauma: it is painful and not very nice. It can be overwhelming to accept the level of trauma present. If we find ourselves thinking of discharging someone without any intervention offered, we need to be aware that this could be part of the picture.

People with ID can be prevented by their families or carers from attending hospital to visit relatives, even attending funerals. This is in a misguided attempt to protect the individual; however, it can bring about more harm. My colleague told me of a someone who saw his mother die at home, when she was rushed to hospital, this person, who had an intellectual disability, was not allowed to go and see her, unlike the rest of his family. Afterwards he sought help to talk about this as he was re-experiencing the death and felt excluded by his family and that they had not been good enough.

Valerie Sinason argues that ID itself is a psychological trauma whether realised or not by the individual. Society is not set up for the disabled individual, who always needs support, who struggles to understand, stands outside, feels other. Also, for the family who struggles to cope with the extra demands there are ripple effects which can lead to them becoming a traumatised family. This has also been seen in a more recent study (McNally, Taggart and Shevlin, 2021).

Re-traumatisation

In one study already discussed, of those people with ID who suffered a trauma in adulthood, half had also had a traumatic event in childhood. Of those who experienced trauma in childhood, all of them suffered another trauma in adulthood (Mason-Roberts et al., 2018). Some symptoms of recurrent traumatisation or trauma in early childhood can be not knowing how to keep yourself safe, not knowing who to trust, possibly being more susceptible to grooming type behaviours, or love bombing (which, for example, abusers have been known to use). The trauma in childhood sometimes isn't disclosed until a re-traumatisation in adulthood which then causes significant behavioural or mental health sequalae, more than might be expected from the later trauma, such as retreating into a disability, not speaking at all or becoming completely deaf.

Mental health services can be stigmatised as not doing their jobs, with blame and trauma reverberating through the network. Team members becoming isolated for example. Although I can't talk about individual patients, all these examples above are common in the different areas I have worked in my career and are from real patients with a trauma history.

A new area that is affecting particularly young people with ID is social media, which can cause secondary trauma from watching Tik Tok videos of self-harm and suicide, and can lead to re-enacting and also violence and aggression. There can be a problem distinguishing reality from fantasy and children and young people are particularly vulnerable to peer pressure which can be added via chat functions. In a recent court case, Dr Venugopal, who was an expert witness, had to watch self-harm content and said it affected his sleep after viewing it on Instagram (Norton and Dirnhuber, 2022). These effects are common to us all to a greater or lesser degree, but I would argue a greater degree for those who are neurodivergent or have an ID, who might start to see these as normal ways of behaving, the more they are exposed to this online. Another example is being groomed or tricked into sending naked pictures and the resulting traumatic exposure and not feeling safe, leading to acute mental illness.

Treatment in ID

Therapy can get very stuck as clients can't remember what was talked about from week to week. Techniques may need to be modified: video or audio recording of key points listened to from week to week can be helpful, as can writing letters or a card with appointment dates, especially around breaks.

People with and without ID can dissociate their bodily pain when they have a history of trauma, having learnt to dissociate to deal with the trauma in childhood. This is known as somatic dissociation. I had one patient who limped and had to start using a wheelchair. An x-ray said there was no pathology in the leg she was protecting by limping. A physiotherapist fortunately realised the issue was coming from the other leg. There was some difficulty getting a second x-ray via the GP but it confirmed that this leg, which she had been weight bearing on, was actually the broken one. How is this possible? She had a long history of trauma as a young woman and child, and trauma had affected her ability to feel her body.

I had another patient who, when she was trying to self-harm, would eye gouge. We became adept at realising she had a physical health issue, recurrent UTI or chest infection. When successfully treated with antibiotics, her self-harm disappeared.

Conversely to dissociation, anxiety can be high in the network supporting the person with ID and complexity, bringing them to the attention of services. Often, they have been through services and everything that is on offer and therapeutic nihilism can be the result. Often the trauma history is not at the forefront of the formulation. Instead, the person with ID might be in crisis with self-harming behaviour, suicidal behaviours, disinhibition. In some people, behaviours which transfer a sense of disgust into the onlooker can be at the forefront, such as smearing faeces. Sexual offending behaviours including in public can be the presenting complaint to professionals.

Sometimes in one or two cases there are alleged and actual offences by carers, sometimes substantiated and sometimes not. People become a subject of safeguarding procedures which results nearly always with support workers leaving or being dismissed, and then working in pairs becoming a norm. Although support staff still report feeling stress and worry that they will lose their job, at the same time they are put at risk of injury and being attacked, especially in situations such as personal care which can be a high-risk time.

The person with ID may feel they might be hurt (due to trauma history) and so can attack first if you like; nearly always this can lead to a high turnover of support workers and sometimes placement breakdowns. Trauma resonates outwards in the network in these cases and it can be the role of the consultant to start to put the bigger picture together and start treating all the layers separately, one by one.

One issue can be repeated allegations against staff which turn out to be false. Working closely with the network and a good social worker and team is key to develop protocols around this so that staff are not suspended and turnover isn't high, all the while ensuring safeguarding of the person with ID by having a local protocol for investigating the allegations, which is signed off by the network. In this way placements can become safe places. People who are traumatised might prefer to have two carers and have less anxiety although these packages of care are more expensive and can impact on number of outings and events.

In terms of treatment, Skelly (2016) advocates for physical safety for the person with ID before any treatment can begin, so a move to a placement which can be tested and can hold is key. Often this is not the case for people that we work with and so repeated placement breakdowns or hospitalisation can occur. People can be left with recreating the sense of not feeling safe and not being able to make progress in their lives.

The other issue can be that some people with ID ring 999 continuously. This can be very problematic as services are obliged to respond. A capacity assessment is needed around understanding the consequences of ringing 999 and why it might be necessary to call that number at times of emergency. Sometimes they do understand and yet still call 999. I have been involved with several patients who have done this and it can be quite difficult. You need meetings with paramedics, GPs, ambulance services and police to agree protocols and ways forward. There is no magic wand you can wave over this except to explain the traumatic background as to why they ring. Simultaneously they are also at higher risk of more severe physical health problems and admission to hospital say once or twice a year. Indeed, pneumonia or something else could genuinely lead to the need for hospitalisation. It is a difficult area that needs to be looked into more carefully. Some places have their own protocols. The ambulance services, for instance. Some individuals who ring constantly without any basis can even be prosecuted. It can lead to conviction and a criminal record.

Conclusion

In summary people with ID are in a high-risk group for developing PTSD should they suffer trauma. They also suffer more ACEs, more life events as an adult and also more trauma in general, the effects of which can accumulate. They have more life-threatening illnesses, bereavements and have memory difficulties which might make processing trauma more difficult. As clinicians not only do we often fail to diagnose PTSD, we often don't even think of trauma as an underlying mediating factor. Sometimes chronicity of the events plays a part in stopping us from thinking of it. However, I wonder also if the sheer weight of the difficulties becomes overwhelming and makes it so that we dissociate from the trauma ourselves, in a sense suffering secondary and tertiary trauma.

At the end of one year a psychiatric junior doctor who was a great doctor and very reflective and self-aware, said what she had learnt working with me was not to be afraid of people with ID anymore. She had never mentioned this at the beginning of the year. It can be overwhelming to work with such levels of complexity and often initially people are referred with challenging behaviour, violence and aggression, which can be worrying for junior doctors and a source of fear. Do we need to do more about this? Do we need to be helping younger people in our professions to feel safe and held?

Or is there something about Alan Corbett's othering (Corbett 1996)? Instead of seeing people with ID as on one end of the human continuum, they are made other.

People with ID are more susceptible to mental health problems, epilepsy, multiple trauma and life events, more physical illness and life-threatening illness, more bereavements and die 16–20 years earlier than those without ID. Does that make them a bit scary to work with? How do you deal with the pain and the overwhelming difficulties?

The main thing I have learnt is that PTSD does not supersede other diagnoses as often these are in addition. In fact, if there is just CPTSD you have probably missed a mental illness, a physical illness in addition. Look again.

In these complex cases, I believe quality of life is the main target outcome and the analogy of aggregation of marginal gains used in cycling (Harrell, 2015) is useful around treatment in CPTSD and people with multiple and complex problems and diagnoses. I first heard this mentioned at a lecture about treatment-resistant depression, however for any population where there is complexity, aggregation of marginal gains is a helpful way of avoiding therapeutic nihilism and, as Sir Dave Brailsford says, it can create an atmosphere of contagious enthusiasm where everyone is looking at ways to improve. Thus, it is worth pursuing.

On one occasion, I was working with someone who probably had complex PTSD. They had been through forensic services so did fit into that pattern of presenting with violence in early life but had never discussed their trauma. I had known them for about five years and had two medical students with me when suddenly all the traumatic childhood history was coming out for the first time when speaking to the students. At first, I was just really glad and felt a sense of relief, that they could speak about this. I had given a diagnosis of PTSD on the basis of symptoms, without a disclosure of a history of trauma. Immediately after I then worried about the medical students, as hearing about people's trauma histories can cause secondary traumatisation in the clinician as previously discussed, particularly as this trauma was quite graphic and gruesome. I checked in with them after the consultation had ended, explained what might happen and checked that they had my contact details in case they did experience any difficulties. I also needed to say that would be an expected reaction as it was detailed information that was given. The good thing was that I felt the person with ID was ready to start again with therapy. It is always good to find a time that is right for therapy to start or start again. So, this did feel the right time for psychotherapy input and they did do very well and improved quite a lot. One of the consequences of the trauma was falling out with neighbours and having to move a lot. These behaviours affect someone's whole life and it can be quite difficult to achieve stability in the person's life. But it is always worth offering therapy again.

In Symington's (1981) classic paper of psychotherapy of a man with ID, the patient did really well. In light of this in his reflection on the therapy, Symington asks himself should he have offered more? Why didn't he? He could have offered a more intensive therapy over longer time? Could the patient have done even better? What held him back from offering this? Was fear a component? Now you have read this chapter you can postulate your own answers to his questions.

PTSD (ICD 10, WHO 2004):

- History of a traumatic event
- Problems with sleep/nightmares
- Flashbacks/re-experiencing
- Jumpiness, agitation/hypervigilance
- Avoidance of triggers/trauma
- Effects on quality of life
- Functional impairments

Complex PTSD (ICD 11, WHO 2018):

- Above PTSD symptoms and:
- Three disturbances of self-organisation:
- Emotional dysregulation
- Interpersonal difficulties
- Negative self-concept

PTSD and CPTSD symptoms in people with intellectual disability:

- Aggression, anger, challenging behaviour
- Sleep problems
- Distractibility

- Distress
- Self-harm
- Social isolation
- Functional effects
- Sexually inappropriate behaviours (Sobsey and Mansell 1994; Mansell, Sobsey and Calder, 1992)
- Poor sense of personal safety, low self-esteem (Mansell, Sobsey and Moskal, 1998)
- Dissociative non-epileptic seizures
- Multiple safe-guarding
- Repeated allegations against staff, which turn out to be false resulting in needing two staff to one patient at all times to prevent high staff turnover
- Calling 999 repeatedly
- More often the history of a traumatic event is absent—possibly due to length of time needed for a trusting relationship, chronicity between the event and the time of symptoms
- Change of behaviour from baseline
- Anxiety in the network
- Dissociation in the network

Bibliography

Bakken, T. L., Kildahl, A. N., Gjersoe, V., et al. (2014). Identification of PTSD in adults with intellectual disabilities in five patients in a specialised psychiatric inpatient unit. *Advances in Mental Health and Intellectual Disability*, 8(2), 91–102.

Barkley, R. A., Murphy, K. R., & Fischer, M. (2008). *ADHD in adults: What the science says*. The Guilford Press.

Brewin, C. R., Rumball, F. and Happa, F. (2019). *Neglected causes of Post-Traumatic Stress Disorder. British Medical Journal.* 365.

Breuer, J. and Freud, S. (1893). On The Psychical Mechanism of Hysterical Phenomena. *The Standard Edition of the Complete Psychological Works of Sigmund Freud*, Volume II. London: The Hogarth Press.

Buckles, J., Luckasson, R. and Keefe, E. (2013). A Systematic Review of the Prevalence of Psychiatric Disorders in Adults with Intellectual Disability, 2003–2010. *Journal of Mental Health Research in Intellectual Disabilities*, 6(3), 181–207.

Byrne, G. (2018). Prevalence and psychological sequelae of sexual abuse among individuals with an intellectual disability: A review of the recent literature. *Journal of Intellectual Disabilities*, 22(3), 294–310.

Cloitre, M. (2020). ICD-11 complex post-traumatic stress disorder: Simplifying diagnosis in trauma populations. *The British Journal of Psychiatry*, 216(3), 129–131.

Corbett A. (1996). *Witnessing, Nurturing, Protesting: Therapeutic Responses to Sexual Abuse of People with Learning Disabilities.* David Fulton Publishers.

Daveney, J. Matcham, F. Sen, P. Hassiotis, A. and Katona, C. (2019). Ascertainment and prevalence of Post-Traumatic Stress Disorder (PTSD) in people with intellectual disabilities. *Journal of Mental Health Research in Intellectual Disabilities*, 12 (3–4), 211–233.

De Vries G.-J. and Olff, M. (2009). The lifetime prevalence of traumatic events and posttraumatic stress disorder in the Netherlands. *Journal of Traumatic Stress*, 22(4): 259–267.

Deb, S., Thomas, M. and Bright, C. (2001). Mental disorder in adults with intellectual disability. Prevalence of functional psychiatric illness among a community-based population aged between 16 and 64 years. *Journal of Intellectual Disability Research*, 45(6), 495–505.

Felitti, V. J., Anda, R. F., Nordenberg, D., Williamson, D. F., Spitz, A. M., Edwards, V., Koss, M. P. and Marks, J. S. (1998). Relationship of Childhood Abuse and Household Dysfunction to Many of the Leading Causes of Death in Adults. The Adverse Childhood Experiences (ACE) Study. *American Journal of Preventative Medicine*, 14(4), 245–258.

Hall, J. C., Jobson, L. & Langdon, E. P. (2014). Measuring symptoms of post-traumatic stress disorder in people with intellectual disabilities: The development and psychometric properties of the Impact of Event Scale-Intellectual Disabilities (IES-IDs). *British Journal of Clinical Psychology*, 53(3), 315–332.

Harrel, E. (2015). How 1% improvement led to Olympic Gold. *Harvard Business Review*, October 30.

Herman, J. L. (1992). Complex PTSD: A syndrome in survivors of prolonged and repeated trauma. *Journal of Traumatic Stress*, 5(3), 377–391.

Hollins, S. & Sinason, V. (2000) Psychotherapy, learning disabilities and trauma: new perspectives. *Br. J. Psychiatry*, 176, 32–36.

Hughes, K., Bellis, M. A., Hardcastle, K. A., Sethi, D., Butchart, A., Mikton, C., Jones L. and Dunne, M. P. (2017). The effect of multiple adverse childhood experiences on health: a systematic review and meta-analysis. *The Lancet*, 2(8), e356–e366.

Karatzias, T., Cloitre, M., Maercker, A., Kazlauskas, E., Shevlin, M., Hyland, P., Bisson, J. I., Roberts, N. P. & Brewin, C. R., (2017a). PTSD and Complex PTSD: ICD-11 updates on concept and measurement in the UK, USA, Germany and Lithuania. *European Journal of Psychotraumatology*, 8(7), 1418103.

Karatzias, T., Shevlin, M., Fyvie, C., Hyland, P., Efthymiadou, E., Wilson, D., Roberts, N., Bisson, J. I., Brewin, C. R. and Cloitre, M. (2017b). Evidence of distinct profiles of Post Traumatic Stress Disorder (PTSD) and Complex Posttraumatic Stress Disorder (CPTSD) based on the new ICD-11 Trauma Questionnaire (ICD-TQ). *J. Affect Disord.*, Jan 1; 207, 181–187.

Kessler, R. C., Berglund, P., Demler, O., Jin, R., Merikangas, K. R. and Walters, E. E. (2005). Lifetime prevalence and age-of-onset distributions of DSM-IV disorders in the National Comorbidity Survey Replication. *Archives of General Psychiatry*, 62 (6), 593–602.

Lanius, R. A., Vermetten, E., Loewenstein, R.J., Brand, B., Schmahl, C., Bremner, J. D. and Spiegel, D. (2010) Emotion modulation in PTSD: Clinical and neurobiological evidence for a dissociative subtype. *Am. J. Psychiatry*, Jun; 167(6), 640–647.

Macklin, M. L., Metzger, L. J., Litz, B. T., McNally, R. J., Lasko, N. B., Orr, S. P. and Pitman, R. K. (1998). Lower precombat intelligence is a risk factor for posttraumatic stress disorder. *Journal of Consulting and Clinical Psychology*, 66(2), 323–326.

Mason-Roberts, S., Bradley, A., Karatzias, T., Brown, M., Paterson, D. R., Walley R., Truesdale M., Taggart, L., & Sirisena, C. (2018). Multiple traumatisation and subsequent psychopathology in people with intellectual disabilities and DSM 5 PTSD: a preliminary study. *JIDR*, 62(8), 730–736.

Matheson, C. (2016). A new diagnosis of complex Post-traumatic Stress Disorder, PTSD – a window of opportunity for the treatment of patients in the NHS? *Psychoanalytic Psychotherapy*, 30(4), 329–344.

McCarthy, J. (2001). Post-Traumatic Stress Disorder in People with Learning Disability. *Advances in Psychiatric Treatment*, 7, 163–169.

McNally, P., Taggart, L. and Shevlin, M. (2021), *Trauma experiences of people with an intellectual disability and their implications: A scoping review. J. Appl. Res. Intellect. Disabil.*, 34, 927–949.

Mevissen-Renckens, E. H. M. and de Jongh, A. (2010). PTSD and its treatment in people with intellectual disabilities: a review of the literature. *Clinical Psychology Review*, Apr; 30(3), 308–316.

Moss, S. and Patel, P. (1993). The prevalence of mental illness in people with intellectual disability over 50 years of age, and the diagnostic importance of information from carers. *Irish Journal of Psychology*, 14, 110–129.

Parkes, G., Mukherjee, R.A.S., Karagianni, E., Attavar, R., Sinason, V. and Hollins, S. (2007). Referrals to an intellectual disability psychotherapy service in an inner city catchment area – a retrospective case notes study. *Journal of Applied Research in Learning Disability.* 20, 4, 373–378.

Rumball, F. (2019). A Systematic Review of the Assessment and Treatment of Post-traumatic Stress Disorder in Individuals with Autism Spectrum Disorders. *Review Journal of Autism and Developmental Disorders*, 6, 3, 294–324.

Ryan, R. (1994). Post Traumatic Stress Disorder in persons with developmental disorder. *Community Mental Health Journal* 30, 1, 45–55.

Mansell, S., Sobsey, D. and Calder, P. (1992). Sexual abuse treatment for persons with developmental disabilities. *Professional Psychology: Research and Practice*, 23, 404–409.

Mansell, S., Sobsey, D. and Moskal, R. (1998). Clinical findings among sexually abused children with and without developmental disabilities. *Mental Retardation*, 36, 12–22.

Norton, J. & Dirnhuber, J. (2022). We posed as a Tik Tok teen and suicide posts appeared in a matter of minutes. *Daily Mail*, 30th September.

Sinason, V. 2002, Some reflections from twenty years of psychoanalytic work with children and adults with a learning disability. *Disability Studies Quarterly*, 22, 3, 38–45.

Skelly, A. (2016). Maintaining the Bond Working with People Who are Described as Showing Challenging Behaviour Using a Framework Based on Attachment Theory. In Fletcher, H. K., Flood A. and Hare, D. J. (eds), *Attachment in Developmental and Intellectual Disability: A Clinicians Guide to Practice and Research*, pp.104–129. Wiley Blackwell.

Sobsey, D. and Mansell, S. (1994). An international perspective on patterns of sexual assault and abuse of people with disabilities. *International Journal of Adolescent Medicine and Health*, 7, 2, 153–178.

Sullivan, P. M. and Knutson, J. F. (2000). The prevalence of disabilities and maltreatment among runaway children. *Child Abuse & Neglect*, 24(10), 1275–1288.

Symington, N. (1981). The psychotherapy of a subnormal patient. *The British Journal of Medical Psychology*, 54, 187–199.

Turk, J., Robbins, I. and Woodhead, M. (2005). Post-traumatic stress disorder in young people with intellectual disability. *Journal of Intellectual Disability Research*, 49, 872–875.

Van der Put, C. E., Asscher, J. J., Wissink, I. B. and Stams, G. J. J. M. (2014). The relationship between maltreatment victimisation and sexual and violent offending:

differences between adolescent offenders with and without intellectual disability. J. Intellect. Disabil. Res., 58, 979–991.

Wigham, S., Hatton, C. and Taylor, J. L. (2011). The Lancaster and Northgate Trauma Scales (LANTS): the development and psychometric properties of a measure of trauma for people with mild to moderate intellectual disabilities. *Research in Developmental Disabilities*, 32(6), 2651–2659.

World Health Organization. 2004. *International Statistical Classification of Diseases and Related Health Problems (10th Revision).* Volume 2, Second Edition.

World Health Organization. 2018. *International Statistical Classification of Diseases and Related Health Problems (11th Revision).* Google Scholar.

Chapter 10

Relationship, Imagination, Justice and Hope

Throughlines in Child Psychotherapy, Trauma, Learning Disability and Social Exclusion

Tamsin Cottis

In November 1982 I attended an event at Mencap headquarters in Golden Lane. The previous summer I had volunteered on Mencap's residential holidays scheme, spending a week at an adventure centre in North Wales with a group of 16 children and adolescents with learning disabilities, among other volunteers from around the UK. We had been sea-kayaking, rock climbing, to the funfair at Barmouth and to Harlech Castle. This reunion in Golden Lane was a chance for Mencap to say thank you to the volunteers for helping. As part of the event, a group of students with learning disabilities, from a new department at the City Lit Adult Education Institute in central London, had been invited to give a short performance of their work. I watched as a small group of adults with and without learning disabilities, led by dancer and choreographer Wolfgang Stange, showed us a contemporary dance they had co-created. The late Harvey Waterman, then in his forties, strummed on a guitar. Harvey spoke to the group and told us he had recently moved back to Hackney after living for nearly four decades in a long stay hospital for people with what was then called 'mental handicap.'

'I like it better in Hackney,' he said, in his quiet voice, 'I can ride the bus to my music class.'

That day, something clicked between me and this group. A few days later, I arranged to join in the Wednesday dance class with Wolfgang. I liked it so much I became a regular member of the class. Through attending classes at City Lit, I realised that the students were often better dancers and more natural musicians than me. We were all learning alongside each other. It was fun, moving and enlightening. I did not feel so much like the 'helper' and 'the person *without* difficulties' as I had through my volunteering. The impact on me was profound.

After a year, as I graduated from my politics degree, Jan Wyatt, the programme director at City Lit, asked if I'd like to join the teaching team.

'But what would I teach?' I said, 'I'm not a dancer or a musician.'

DOI: 10.4324/9781003646242-14

I knew Jan felt strongly that people with learning disabilities should be taught by experts; their tuition should be top class. It's a view I've been influenced by when arguing for quality therapy for people with learning disabilities, over the years.

'You know about politics,' she said. 'Do that.'

The idea seemed outlandish but I was encouraged and emboldened by Jan's enthusiasm. Later, this *'Give it a go'* mentality, found a reflection in the way we went about setting up Respond, and developing our model of disability psychotherapy there, when it was Valerie Sinason and Anne Craft and Sheila Hollins who encouraged and supported us.

I began to teach a group at City Lit where we talked about politics, and the world around us. We went on visits to the Old Bailey, to the Houses of Parliament – to meet sympathetic MPs and for students to voice their views. The London Transport Museum was also a favourite place: the free travel, and the liberating network of underground trains and buses seemed to be the embodiment of the freshly granted freedom the students had, now out of hospital and back in the London districts where they'd spent their childhoods, and to which they felt deep attachment.

In our classes, the students talked about their lives and shared their past and present lived experiences. This included Harvey, with whom I would go on to work as both teacher and colleague for many years. He became an actor, and a sought-after self-advocate, right up to his death aged 82 in 2020. He talked in short quiet sentences, about life in the hospital, learning to use the buses and tubes, getting a free travel pass, but wanting the stigmatising orange 'H' for 'Handicapped' that was printed on it, to be removed.

The self-advocacy movement was in its infancy in the early 1980s in the UK but we at City Lit jumped on board. We held and attended conferences where people talked about being free to make their own choices; their equal rights as people to live with who they wanted to, to live where they chose. These were heady times and I was full of political zeal.

As the discussion groups matured, the students in them talked about their more difficult experiences too, especially in terms of relationships. I began to realise that the students wanted what most people – including me – wanted: to love and be loved and be free to express themselves verbally, emotionally, physically, sexually. We talked more about this in the group. Lynda told us how hard it had been to persuade the staff in her group home to get her a double bed, for example. She wanted to sleep with her boyfriend John, also a resident.

The students also began to talk about the bad sexual things that had happened to them.

Margaret, now in her 50s said, 'In the hospital, the men just did what they felt like doing to you. There was nothing you could really do about it. The staff never took no notice.'

She sounded sad, and resigned more than angry. But her friend, Elizabeth, was still furious about the member of hospital staff who sexually abused her and made her pregnant,

'They took my daughter away from me. I never even got to hold her!'

At that time, the late 1980s, there was a lot of talk in British society about child sexual abuse. Historic scandals within the Catholic Church, and local authority children's homes were beginning to come to light. It became clear that people with learning disabilities had also been vulnerable. And still were.

Among colleagues in the self-advocacy movement were a number of people who, like me, faced the issue of supporting people who'd been abused, and we felt ill-equipped, shocked and somewhat traumatised, by what we were hearing. We had thought we were supporting people in their rights to enjoy sexual freedom. It turned out many needed support in facing down painful memories and experiences from the past. I remember running a 'sex and relationships' group for women with learning disabilities. I took in anatomical pictures of adults: so many people I'd worked with had such very hazy basic knowledge about sex and the body. At the sight of an image of a naked man, however, several women became distressed and left the room in tears. How naïve and foolish I felt. Guilty, too, for being insensitive.

In the early 1990s I teamed up with two others who felt as I did about these issues: Steve Morris and Alan Corbett. We had an idea for an organisation, or network of some kind, generated from discussions round our kitchen tables. We wanted to link up with other people who, like us, were supporting survivors of sexual abuse who had learning disabilities. Respond was started. For the next ten years or so, we were supported and encouraged by others in this field, notably Valerie Sinason, the late Professor Ann Craft and Professor – later, Baroness – Sheila Hollins. Respond grew from an idea for a support and training service to a counselling and psychotherapy service, running groups and individual sessions for people with learning disabilities who had been sexually abused. We also provided training and seminars for staff from a range of organisations and joined campaigns to reduce the vulnerability of people with learning disabilities to abuse of all kinds.

In the early days of Respond there was a lot of overlap with the self-advocacy I'd been doing. In many ways, the work we wanted to do was driven by a commitment to equality, and for creating opportunities for people with learning disabilities to be seen and heard, even when what they were saying was very hard to hear, and challenging of services. But we also began to realise the depth of emotional distress that was inside people; and crucially how much so-called 'challenging behaviour' that people with learning disabilities displayed, in fact had traumatic, unwitnessed, unacknowledged experiences of abuse at its root. Of course, Valerie Sinason's groundbreaking work was instrumental here (Sinason, 1992).

We wanted to find out more about what people had been through; to provide some witnessing, empathy and understanding. If we didn't work to find out more about what had happened to people, to help them, and their carers, and make those links between past and present, then an injustice was being perpetrated. After all, other people got therapy in the wake of abuse – why not people with learning disabilities?

In terms of alerting us to the issue, and in providing therapeutic support, and in bringing concerned staff and supporters together, Valerie was the pioneer – running the Mental Handicap Workshop at the Tavistock, being personally and professionally supportive to us at Respond. We were not qualified psychotherapists and were very much finding our way into this complicated, painful world. As well, we got policy and financial support from the government of the time, and started up the steep learning curve of fundraising and budgeting. Donors, such as Comic Relief, were also vital early supporters.

As we got more involved, we discovered that some of the people who been abused, were in turn a sexual risk to others. There was no specific service addressing their needs for treatment and support. Their rights were often undefended and freedoms denied as they were put under 24-hour supervision with no framework for interrogating the length of time that such restrictions would be in place. This development into working with perpetrators of abuse was a very challenging one for me. But rejecting the simple victim/perpetrator split was reflective of our wish not to see things in simple either/or terms. All people are a complicated mix of good and bad. All of us have the potential to hate and hurt as well as love and nurture.

I think I already understood (from difficulties in my own childhood as well as through my work choices) that our lived experience profoundly influences the things we do, and – in particular –the kinds of relationships we form, and how we treat other people. I see this in my work today with children who are getting on so badly with all the people in their lives, as well as themselves. And I saw it then in some of the people with learning disabilities – usually, but not always, men, whose behaviour was a danger to others. Their victim experiences were generally not hard to recognise, especially if one was open to them.

In the formative years of Respond the small group of staff spent many hours talking about these things – ideas and themes which felt philosophical, political, historical, as well as connected to the most effective ways to develop and deliver therapy. It was very much a process of learning by doing and the support of others outside this small group was essential.

The government changed in 1997 and in 2000 the UK signed up to the European Human Rights Act (Human Rights Act, 1998). Equality as human beings was now enshrined in law. Then, Valuing People (Department of Health 2001) the new government policy on services for people with learning disabilities put the service users' voice at the heart of its policy-making (though sadly the money didn't follow the good intentions for long). The policy document containing and representing the views of families was called, '*Nothing About Us Without Us.*'

Additionally, the law regarding sexual offences had for many decades been stacked against the safety of people with learning disabilities. Along with Voice UK and the Ann Craft Trust and many others, Respond took part in a review of the Sexual Offences Act (UK Government, 2003). By the time the new Act was published in 2004, the Memorandum of Good Practice (Home Office, 1992) which set out new procedures for investigating allegations of abuse had also been amended to help ensure that, if a case involving the sexual offence against a person learning disability did come to court, they would be supported in their fight for justice by provisions or 'Special Measures' (Department of Health, 2001) for victims deemed as 'vulnerable.' Such measures had previously only existed for children, leaving learning-disabled witnesses to crimes on their own, and open to damaging cross examination in criminal courts. The changes in law meant that people in positions of responsibility were also less free to act with impunity. The Criminal Records Bureau (now the Disclosure and Barring Service) introduced comprehensive checks, meaning that staff found responsible for acts of sexual abuse or criminality could not simply stay in their posts, or be redeployed elsewhere, as we knew from the testimony of our service users had been happening up to this point.

A lot of these positive changes have proved less than perfect in reality, and a shortfall in funding to make sure they are delivered on the ground has been a constant pretty much ever since. Sometimes the gap between stated intention and reality seems depressingly wider every day. But as statements of value and intent they seemed significant at the time, and we were proud at Respond to be even a small part of bringing the changes about.

This was also, crucially, the time that the Institute for Psychotherapy and Disability (IPD) was formed. I was getting more and more interested in the practice and process of psychotherapy itself. The roots of our therapeutic model at Respond were in psychoanalysis. With Valerie's clinical guidance, along with that of Sheila Hollins, we came to understand the power of unconscious communications, projection and the process of transference.

Additionally, we saw more clearly how fear and hatred of 'the other' lay in a 'social unconscious' that devalued the lives of people with learning disabilities, also reviled because – in a hyper-capitalist society – their economic worth was negative. Dr Earl Hopper was a staunch educator and supporter at this time too. I came to see that the perceived low value of learning-disabled lives may be a factor on the hate crime they experience, their difficulties accessing adequate medical care and their vulnerability to abuse within institutions set up to provide housing and care (Mencap, 2010, 2012; Ryan, 2018; Hopper, 1997), including in gaining equal access to mental health services.

I don't remember people talking about 'structural inequality' and 'systemic discrimination' in those days, but I can see now that's what we were working with. We worked to develop Respond as a centre of excellence for psychotherapy for people with learning disabilities, engaging in further training ourselves, as well as running courses and workshops for other professionals, including psychotherapists who were not experienced with people with learning disabilities. I talked of this as an equality issue. If people generally had a right to good quality psychotherapy, then so did people with learning disabilities. And if the 'mainstream' treatment options available were not a good fit for the particular needs of people with learning disabilities then it was incumbent on practitioners to be creative and open to change in order to find ways to engage and make relationships. The IPD was advocating fiercely for such changes in understanding and practice.

Through the early 2000s, Respond began to work with learning-disabled adolescents, and then children. Art and dance therapists joined our team. Toys and art materials were introduced to the therapy rooms. In my own practice, the work of Winnicott, with his understanding of the lifelong significance of creativity and play in being able to be our fullest selves became increasingly important. As the theoretical foundations of our work widened, and our services increased, in 2009, we produced a book about our work at Respond (Cottis, 2009). Noelle Blackman, Richard Curen and David O'Driscoll had joined Respond, increasing our expertise in working with offenders, in the field of loss and bereavement and with the often uncharted histories of people with learning disabilities, such as Harvey, who had been confined to institutions for decades (Curen, 2009; Blackman, 2003; O'Driscoll, 2009).

Development and growth as an organic, evolving process, with a creative relationship at its heart, has been one of the throughlines of my working life. It has melded my early experience as a teenage volunteer, getting involved at City Lit, at Respond, and continued all the way through to now, in my role as a child psychotherapist.

Over the years, at Respond and in my training as an integrative child psychotherapist, I have developed a theoretical underpinning to my practice (Cottis, 2021). It has a number of core elements. These include Attachment Theory (Bowlby, 1953) and Winnicottian object relations, including the significance of transitional objects (Winnicott, 1984). Anne Alvarez's work, (1992, 2012) has also been highly significant to my understanding and practice of psychotherapy. Her work is rooted in Object Relations Theory and brings us the concept of the therapist as 'live company' (Alvarez, 1992) and her profoundly important framework the 'Levels of Working' (Alvarez, 2010). Alvarez puts the power of relationship firmly at the centre of her psychoanalytic practice with hard-to-reach and disturbed children.

Another key influence has been Dan Hughes's PACE model (Hughes, 2007), which has playfulness, acceptance, curiosity and empathy at its core. I have also come to understand that art, creativity and play are essential to the development of a secure sense of self. I work with a sensibility of the ways in which the impact of trauma including neglect, and other forms of abuse, has long-reaching and profound effects on the nervous system (van der Kolk,

2014); a system in which mind and body are indivisible. I also recognise more strongly than ever that what has *happened* to people, and what societal structures do to them will affect how they feel about themselves, and how they behave. The work of psychologists, trauma specialists and neuroscientists such as Allan Schore, (1994) Bessell van der Kolk (2005), Bruce Perry, (2006) and Stephen Porges (2011) has helped us find ways to reach those whose difficult experiences have affected their brain development. Van der Kolk's model of Developmental Trauma (2005) shows how persistent traumatic experiences affect every aspect of a child's functioning, including their capacity to trust others, and to be able to relax into the emotional state which makes being happily with another person a safe, rewarding, reciprocally enriching experience. Learning and cognitive development are also adversely affected by traumatic experience, and the work regarding the impact of Adverse Childhood Experiences (ACEs) (Hughes et al., 2017) has helped bring this clearly into public understanding. Again, Alvarez's work, and that of Valerie Sinason, in particular her work on 'secondary handicap' (1992) has been pivotal in deepening our understanding and practice in such circumstances.

February 2022

Belle (some details have been changed to protect anonymity) is in her therapy session. She is thwacking an inflatable globe hard against the therapy room wall, listing all the things that make her angry, 'Unfair teachers, my annoying sister, boring work, rubbish internet, not having my own phone, girls who you thought were friends and now you can't trust them.'

Aged 10, Belle is the second of three children, in Year 6 at her local primary school. While Belle was in Year 5, her parents' marriage broke up. Her father returned to Nigeria, following allegations of violence towards her mother. Belle, who is very able academically, has been unhappy and angry since then. She is disruptive in lessons and regularly in trouble for instigating arguments, making cruel comments and sometimes having physical fights, with other girls. There have been a lot of difficulties with friendships in the class, and Belle often has to sit by herself in lessons. She has had two fixed-term exclusions for fighting, and a number of internal exclusions. She has forfeited many breaktimes due to behaviour which risks the well-being and safety of others. She is defiant and rude to her teacher, walking out of class, kicking over furniture. Belle has told a teaching assistant who has known her for many years that her mother favours her younger brother and that she misses her father, 'even though he got mad at us sometimes.'

Belle has been seeing me for weekly therapy sessions for the past two school terms. I have found the work demanding. She has a kind of brittle bravado, which means that acknowledging feelings of fear, or vulnerability, is extremely difficult for her. She has hardly talked directly about her home circumstances. She refers occasionally to fights with her siblings but does not talk about either of her parents. I understand the prior involvement of social services has made her wary of disclosing information which may bring unwelcome safeguarding interventions.

I think Belle also doesn't talk about her parents because she is protecting herself from the feelings of sadness and vulnerability that will follow if she is open about the pressures and losses she has faced and continues to face.

I am passionate about using play, art and metaphor to support children to express both their feelings and their experiences. I know I need to handle Belle's vulnerabilities with tenderness and respect. I am also acutely aware that Belle's challenging social and economic circumstances are part of the difficulties she currently faces.

I can see many connections between my work with Belle and my previous work as a therapist, working at Respond, with adults and young people with learning disabilities:

1   Belle finds it hard to express herself directly with words, and the therapy cannot rely only on her narrative accounts of how she is feeling, and what has happened to her.
2   Her social, economic circumstances and her place in society as a girl of colour is relevant to how she feels about the world and herself in it.
3   My role as therapist is connected with other people who are concerned with Belle – her family, the Special Educational Needs Coordinator (SENCO) and teachers at school, the Safeguarding Officer and the family's social worker. The work is taking place in a private space but it cannot offer complete confidentiality, and Belle will be better served if the adults around her are able to work productively together, although we have different roles in, and views about, her situation.

The feelings Belle has brought to sessions are mainly her anger, and also a smouldering sense of injustice. Belle presents as outgoing, outspoken, defiant, unconcerned about other people and unafraid of getting into trouble with authority. Finding ways to both witness and respect these emotional experiences whilst also supporting her to feel safe enough to express a wider range of feelings, including sadness, vulnerability or shame has been difficult.

'I'm fine, I'm good,' she often says, arms folded against her chest. 'It's just I keep getting blamed for things I didn't do. It's *so* unfair and of course I don't like it. So I try to be calm but I get angry. Teachers say fighting is wrong, but if someone says bad things about my family, I'm not going to just let that go, am I?'

Today, she asks if we can play Jenga. I have written questions on the bricks. One question says, '*If I had three wishes I would…*'

'I'd get an iPhone 11, a new laptop and make a law against unfair teachers,' she says.

Next, she pulls out, '*I get frustrated when…*'

Belle answers, 'I get frustrated when adults fight and don't care about how the kids feel.'

'That is hard when that happens,' I say, using a strong voice, 'That *shouldn't* happen to children. If you heard about that happening to kids, what would you want to say to the adults?'

'Dunno,' she shrugs, 'Maybe something like, "We've got feelings too, you know!"'

'You're right about that, Belle,' I say. 'For sure.'

Belle pulls out a supporting brick from the base of the tower and it crashes loudly to the table top. She shouts, 'Yesssss!'

Strong responses, where Belle's own circumstances don't have to be mentioned directly, and which play to her sense of injustice, rather than sadness or vulnerability, seem to be easier for her to accept. Her voice is calmer as she picks up the inflatable globe again.

'Can I tell you something, Miss?'

'Of course,' I say.

She starts thwacking the ball against the wall.

'Just when I got picked for the team, we might have to move house!'

I am so pleased to hear about the team selection: Belle is an excellent footballer, but her angry outbursts have kept her out of the team for several weeks. I am also shocked about the move. 'That's great about the team,' I say. 'Well done. Tell me more about the move.'

Belle keeps on kicking at the ball, head down, 'We're supposed to be playing St Gabriel's next week. They're really good, but Ms Lewis thinks we can beat them.' In her voice I hear a flicker of the will to win.

'I'm sure she's right, Belle. I know she believes in the team and in you.'

Her head stays down.

I find a small light ball, start kicking it myself, beside her, avoiding direct eye contact.

'The landlord's putting our rent up. Mum can't afford it so the council say we have to move. It may be Birmingham. I've never even been to Birmingham! I don't want to go to a new school. *This* is the only school I know! I've been in that house since I was two. My little sister was born there.'

She thwacks the ball hard enough to make me jump back.

The current cap on benefits (UK Government, 2021) puts a ceiling on how much total money in state aid any family can receive, irrespective of size of family or where they live. As a result, many families now find that their London rent is no longer covered by housing benefit. If they are in private rented accommodation, they are especially vulnerable to rent rises. If the benefit threshold is exceeded, they have no option but to become homeless in London or agree to a move to social housing in a different, cheaper area: they are relocated.

As Belle talks, I think what a move would be like for her. Members of staff at her current school are rooting for her, daring to hope she will make it to the Leavers Assembly at the end of Year 6, the day of communal shirt sign-ing, parties and farewell tears: a good ending to her Primary School days.

The school knows Belle and understands the impact of the challenges she has faced. At a new school, she wouldn't even have a whole academic year to make friends; for her and her teachers to get to know each other. The school-based relationships that help keep her more or less on track will be shredded by geo-graphy and circumstances beyond her control. Here, she has a place allocated at the local, familiar secondary school, where her brother is doing ok.

'My mum's so stressed about the move,' Belle says. 'She was crying last night. And that set my little sister off. She's soooo annoying, crying and crying like a baby. My brother was just on his phone. I tried talking to my friends to take my mind off it but then there was a stupid row online and today Ayesha isn't talking to me because Hajra told her I didn't like her. I never said that, so now I hate Hajra. Plus, I forgot my homework so I got put down onto Red because Miss didn't even believe I'd done it.'

'That all sounds very hard,' I say.

'Can we play our wall-tennis,' she says, 'Try and beat our record.'

We often play fast, hard games with the globe. These seem to help Belle discharge energy and aggression. She no longer pretends to throw the globe right in my face, laughing when I flinch, which I understood as a way of putting her fear of sudden attack briefly into someone else.

As the session comes to an end Bella asks if she can draw. I have a set of fifty felt pens that clip together and roll up into a spiral. Belle draws a picture of herself, then a big speech bubble coming out of her month. 'This is what I want to say to the council.' In the bubble she writes, 'I HATE you and I hate my life! You don't even care about us. I DON'T want to go to a new school!'

'I get that Belle,' I say. 'I really, really hope you don't have to move.'

Then she clips the pens together, rolls them up carefully, stacks them safely in their plastic container and presses the lid down firmly, 'There,' she says. 'Safe till next week.'

After Belle has gone back to class I feel my distress acutely. I talk with the school SENCO. She has been supporting Belle in her efforts to manage her angry feelings, arranging some extra support in the class, and for a small group of Year 6 girls to work with a learning mentor on 'Making friends; Staying friends.' The SENCO tells me she will write a letter for Belle's mother, in support of the family's need to stay in the local area. I also con-tribute a short report about Belle – the progress she's made – and the possible impact of a move at this point in her development.

This role of advocate for Belle is also one I am familiar with from my days when my therapy clients were adults and young people with learning dis-abilities, coming to Respond. Many times, decisions were made about where our clients should live, or spend their time, and however strongly they them-selves disagreed with the decision, they were often powerless to stop the changes going ahead.

Belle was referred as a child whose behaviour was a problem – out of line with how the school felt it should be. But she wasn't a list of her behaviours, or of her background, her circumstances as a child of colour, or child growing up in a violent home. She was Belle; her own self. And it was my job to get to know her.

'*How does it feel to be you?*' That's what I wondered when I first met her. It's also what I wondered when I met Cathy, a woman with Down Syndrome, who put her life seriously at risk because she couldn't stop eating.

Cathy came to a Respond group for women who had experienced sexual abuse. A male member of staff at her Day Centre had sexually abused her over a two-year period, coming round to her flat, telling her he loved her and that he would leave his wife for her. He was then discovered to have been abusing a number of women at the Centre, telling each of them they were his 'special one.'

In one group session, Cathy picked up the cloth model of a man we had, punched him, tore at his hair, scratched his cloth face with her fingernails. And then she threw the model out of the window, three floors down to the street below, howling with distress.

'I thought I was special, I thought it was just me!' she screamed at her absent abuser. 'Then I found out you had loads of us. You are disgusting!'

The therapeutic task has, for me, always been to understand what combination of personality and experience has brought this person to the room, now. And how can I understand them better and help them to understand themselves better? For Cathy it was providing the space, scope and empathy to enable her to express her rage and sadness. For Belle it was an inflatable globe, some particular felt pens, time and taking it at her own pace.

Belle was supported by the Special Needs Coordinator in the primary school. Of identified special needs in school age children, 17% are currently needing support because of SEMH – i.e. their social and emotional mental health (Department of Education, 2020). These figures will probably be even higher now, post-COVID and with ever-deepening social and economic inequality.

Belle didn't have learning disabilities like Cathy or Harvey at City Lit, but her emotional difficulties were preventing her from accessing the curriculum; from getting the education that her luckier peers could enjoy. Troubles at home spilled over so that she could not make the most of peer and adult relationships available to her in a caring primary school. Belle's need to present a 'false self' (Winnicott, 1984) to defend against feelings of fear and sadness put her out of tune with herself, shutting off opportunities for full feeling, of being able to experience pleasure and joy in relationships as well as pain. Trauma had impacted her capacity to regulate her emotions, so she would become overwhelmed by rage, and, at times, lash out at others.

Harvey and Cathy were disadvantaged by society's systems; by the low value accorded their lives. I think the same is also true for Belle. A punitive government desire to alter the benefits system pays no regard to her and her family's particular circumstances. It was the same for Harvey, sent away in the early 1940s, as a four-year-old.

There are individual lives and experiences, there are services which can't or won't do the job as well as they know how to – often due to lack of funds – and there are cultural, societally held views about which lives matter most. This was true in the early 1980s and it is true now. In recent years, the Black Lives Matter Movement and #MeToo have shown us this. People with learning disabilities have known it for many, many decades (O'Driscoll, 2009; Cottis, 2018); they cannot be sure that their very lives will be 'allowable.' In 2021, 4.2 million children were living in poverty (Child Poverty Action Group, 2021). A disproportionate number of them were children of colour (Child Poverty Action Group, 2021).

Life chances are being adversely affected by structural decisions within society's systems. I'm as angry about this as I was when I heard about Harvey's separation from his family, or Cathy's abuse and about the failure to prosecute, or even sack, members of staff in learning disability provision who abused those in their care.

Sara Ryan's book (2018) describes the shocking and preventable death of her dearly loved son, Connor Sparrowhawk, in a residential care setting, in 2013. It details her battle with national institutions and public bodies to get recognition of her son's life, a family's loss and systemic failings in care.

It seems the struggle goes on. Where there are inequalities of personhood in societal structures and institutions, there will be a continuing need to protest and campaign for better.

Today, in my work with children, I love to play, and 'see what happens,' creating things from within a containing structure which is firm, yet flexible. When I start working with a child, I am entering a relationship, from the basis of understanding that it is the relationship itself – how we will *be* together, as human beings in a dynamic relationship, as much as what we will *do*, which will do most of the healing work. In this process I am drawing on my training, my experience, my personal politics and my individual personality.

I am, additionally, an agent of hope, saying metaphorically and literally 'By us being together in this room, I believe that things can get better.'

Bibliography

Alvarez, A. (1992). *Live Company*. London: Routledge.
Alvarez, A. (2012). *The Thinking Heart*. London: Routledge.
Blackman. N. (2003). *Loss and Learning Disability*. London: Worth Publishing.
Bowlby, J. (1953). *Child Care and the Growth of Maternal Love*. London. Penguin.
Child PovertyAction Group. (2021). https://cpag.org.uk/child-poverty/child-poverty-facts-and-figures (last accessed 22.11.24).
Child PovertyAction Group. (2021). https://cpag.org.uk/policy-and-campaigns/understanding-and-responding-ethnic-minority-child-poverty#footnote1_s5c00o5 (last accessed 22.11.21).

Cottis, T. (2009) (ed.). *Intellectual Disability, Trauma and Psychotherapy.* London: Routledge.

Cottis, T. (2018). You be the murderer now. In Adlam, J., Kluttig, T. and Lee, B. X. (Eds), *Violent States and Creative States Volume 2: Human Violence and Creative Humanity*, pp.137–149. London: Jessica Kingsley Publications.

Cottis, T. (2021). *How it Feels to Be You: Objects, Play and Child Psychotherapy.* London: Karnac.

Curen, R. (2009). Can they see in the door? Issues in the assessment and treatment of sex offenders who have intellectual disabilities. In Cottis, T. (ed.) *Intellectual Disability, Trauma and Psychotherapy*, pp.90–113. London: Routledge.

Department of Education. (2020). https://www.gov.uk/children-with-special-educational-needs (last accessed 22.01.24).

Department of Health. (2001). Valuing People: A New Strategy for Learning Disability for the 21st Century. https://assets.publishing.service.gov.uk/media/5a7b854740f0b62826a041b9/5086.pdf (accessed 22.01.2024).

Hopper. E. (1997). Traumatic Experience in the Unconscious Life of Groups: A Fourth Basic Assumption. *Group Analysis*, 30(4), 439–470. doi:10.1177/0533316497304002

Hopper, E. (2012). Some Challenges to the Capacity to Think, Link and Hope in the Provision of Psychotherapy for the Learning Disabled. In J. Adlam, A., Aiyegbusi, P., Kleinot, A., Motz, and C. Scanlon, C. (Eds.), *The Therapeutic Milieu under Fire: Security and Insecurity in Forensic Mental Health* (pp. 229–240). London: Jessica Kingsley.

Human Rights Act. (1998). https://www.equalityhumanrights.com/en/human-rights/human-rights-act (last accessed 20.11.21)

Hughes, D. A. (2007). *Attachment-Focused Family Therapy.* New York: W. W. Norton & Co.

Hughes, K., Bellis, M. A., Hardcastle, K. A.*et al.* (2017). The Effect of Multiple Adverse Childhood Experiences on Health: A Systematic Review and Meta-Analysis. *The Lancet*, 2, IssueBPE356–E366.

Home Office. (1992). Memorandum of Good Practice on Video Recorded Interviews with Child Witnesses for Criminal Proceedings.

Mencap. (2010). *Don't Stand By.* https://www.mencap.org.uk/sites/default/files/2016-08/Don%27t%20stand%20by-research-report%20(1).pdf (last accessed 31.1.24).

Mencap (2012). *Death by Indifference; 74 Deaths and Counting.* https://www.mencap.org.uk/sites/default/files/2016-08/Death%20by%20Indifference%20-%2074%20deaths%20and%20counting.pdf (last accessed 31.1.24).

O'Driscoll, D. (2009). Psychotherapy and Intellectual Disability: A Historical View. In Cottis, T. (ed.), *Intellectual Disability, Trauma and Psychotherapy*, pp.9–29. London: Routledge.

Perry, B. (2006). *The Boy Who Was Raised as a Dog.* New York: Basic Books.

Porges, S.W. (2011). *The Polyvagal Theory: Neurophysiological Foundations of Emotions, Attachment, Communication, Self-Regulation.* New York: W.W. Norton & Company.

Ryan, S. (2018). *Justice for Laughing Boy: A Death by Indifference.* London: Jessica Kingsley.

Schore, A. (1994). *Affect Regulation and the Origin of the Self: The Neurobiology of Emotional Development*, Mahwah, NJ: Lawrence Erlbaum Associates.

Sinason, V. (1992). *Mental Handicap and the Human Condition*(First Edition).London: Free Association Books.

UK Government. (2003). *Sex Offences Act.* www.legislation.gov.uk (last accessed 20.11.21).

UK Government. (2021). Benefits Cap. https://www.gov.uk/benefit-cap (last accessed 31.1.24).

Van der Kolk, B. (2005). Developmental Trauma Disorder: Toward a rational diagnosis for children with complex trauma histories. *Psychiatric Annals,* 35(5), 401–408.

Van der Kolk, B. (2014). *The Body Keeps the Score.* London: Penguin.

Winnicott D. W. (1984). *Through Paediatrics to Psychoanalysis.* London: Karnac.

Chapter 11

In Search of Eclecticism as a Means to Navigate the Complexities of Disability Psychotherapy

Nancy Sheppard

In a YouTube video made by a group of young people in the USA who are described by the state as having "special needs", the narrator asks "What are special needs?" The video goes on to explore this question suggesting it would be "special" if people needed to eat dinosaur eggs, wear a suit of armour to the supermarket or be massaged by a cat! The narrator concludes the film with a statement:

"Our needs are not 'Special': what we want is education, jobs, and opportunities, friends and a bit of love – are these needs special?" (March, 2017).

Whether such needs are special has indeed, also posed services with the dilemma of whether to offer specialist services to young people with disabilities or to absorb referrals into mainstream services; similar dilemmas have been debated over the years in education, criminal justice and social services. It is clear, however, despite the efforts of many campaigners and policy makers – seen for instance in the Equalities Act (Department of Health, 2010), Valuing People (Department of Health, 2001), Valuing People Now (Department of Health, 2009), the *Treat Me Right* Campaign (Mencap, 2004), Death by Indifference (Mencap, 2007), Healthcare for all (2008), Closing the Gap Disability Rights Commission (2006), Transforming Care (Department of Health, 2012) – as well as dedicated clinicians (Hadley, Greenhill and Beard [2019]; Bender [1993]), that there is not equal access to services. And, particularly in mental health services, data has shown that people with lower intellectual ability are 25% more likely to complain of symptoms of common mental health problems. Indeed, studies have shown that up to 54% of people with intellectual disabilities have a mental health issue (Cooper et al., 2007). Furthermore, Emerson and Hatton (2007) show that children with intellectual disabilities are 4.5 times more likely to experience mental health difficulties than those without ID. Whittle et al. (2019), on the other hand, focused on identifying barriers that prevent people with intellectual disabilities accessing mental health services, while Chinn and Abraham (2016) note that unequal access to mainstream psychological services remains a dilemma in which specialist services for people with intellectual disabilities could support mainstream services and mobilise towards improving access to emotional support.

DOI: 10.4324/9781003646242-15

It therefore remains important to offer services that make mental health support accessible to children with intellectual disabilities and to neuro-diverse children, as well as their families. Working in a specialist disability Child and Adolescent Mental Health Services (CAMHS) service we are often asked to see young people and their families where other services have felt that their clinical skills have reached their limit and they can no longer help. This has left us thinking carefully about what we do offer and what the specialist nature of our work is.

"Treating with Respect"

In systemic practice it is vital that we understand our own journeys in order to explore the assumptions that we make when faced with other people's stories (Baum and Lynggaard (2006). In Cognitive Analytic Therapy we are encouraged to explore the "Helpers Dance" to gain the understanding that helping is a joint activity, to support us to attune to the patients' experience, and to recognise and name reciprocal roles that might emerge through the therapeutic relationship (Potter, 2014). Every journey has a starting place and in approaching this chapter I have been drawn back to my initial experiences as a young care assistant where I can see myself taking the first steps towards putting down the fundamental roots in value and respect from which my practice has grown.

Working as a care assistant in a hospital for the mentally handicapped I was faced with two entirely different approaches to the work, influenced by the different ward managers that I was working under. On one day making beds, personal care and keeping the ward neat and tidy were the priority, but on the days when Annie our ward manager was there she would sweep in, dressed beautifully, carrying a tray of fresh baked croissants and announce that making the beds could wait as it was coffee and croissants on the terrace for our beautiful ladies. Or she would burst out of the office after a meeting, ask the ladies if we could switch off the TV, put on music, and get us all up and dancing. Annie would book the ward holiday in the grandest hotel that the budget would stretch to and we would have a week of afternoon teas, strolling on the promenade, cocktail hour and themed parties in the evening. I can honestly say this was the best and most fun job I ever had and we truly loved our ladies like they were my own relatives.

This was a powerful lesson in compassion, value and respect, one that was echoed in my first reading of Symington (1992) where he noted the counter-transference feelings of therapists joining the initial Mental Handicap workshop. He describes one therapist admitting that, in getting ready for work and remembering she was only meeting with her intellectually disabled client that day, she would wear her shabby dress rather than the smart one, whilst another member confesses that he attended less to being on time for his intellectually disabled patients than others he saw in the clinic. The Mental Handicap Workshop set up in the 1980s at the Tavistock Centre by Jon Stokes and Valerie Sinason (1992) provided a safe space to name and explore these countertransference feelings of devaluation and allowed the members to transform the experiences of overlooking or dismissing to respectful compassion and thoughtful reflection. Corbett (2019) brought together a number of authors who have described the value of the space that the Mental Handicap Workshop provided and how the forum allowed exploration and thinking about their work which in turn, helped them to undertake effective therapeutic support for people with intellectual disabilities. I was able to join the workshop and experience this first hand and have tried to foster this stance in my work as a clinician, as a supervisor, and as a team manager. I have aimed to support my colleagues to recognise and name difficult feelings and to give voice to them in a safe space in order that respect and compassion are maintained in our work.

Sam brought her work with Sean's parents to supervision. They had been undertaking a functional analysis in order to co-create a positive behaviour support plan to address Sean's angry outbursts. Sam had been feeling increasingly hopeless and had had to brace herself in the face of critical comments about the work and its potential for change. Sam emailed to ask if she could discuss this and came into her supervision saying she thought it might be best if she passed the case to a colleague with more experience than her. We used the supervision session to explore some of the issues Sam had been experiencing and as she was explaining the parent's responses to her suggestions she burst into tears. We took our time, and thought carefully about the material she had brought and the feelings it had stirred up in her. I reminded her about how successful she had been with other families using this model and named some of her qualities in the work that she had been doing in the team. As she relaxed, we were able to tease out what she could recognise as her own anxiety in working with the high achieving couple, who she feared would judge her or might raise a complaint, and what she could see were the family's own insecurities about getting things wrong with their son. She used her supervision to explore the possibilities that the couple were tussling with bearing the pain of realising the extent of Sean's disabilities and even ideas of how this disability might serve as a narcissistic injury to their own egos in the face of their loss of the hoped-for child. Once Sam understood the responses from a position of bearing pain in the parents, and how their responses might be a defence to protect them from feeling they were good enough or had failed in some way in their parenting task, she was able to begin to empathise with their position and attune to their loss. By recognising these countertransference feelings and responding accordingly, Sam was eventually able to name the more painful feelings of hopelessness and loss with the family and the work could progress.

The importance of history, social construction and society's "death wish"

Hodges (2003, p. 5) states that "when considering a person's inner world, it is important to be mindful of not only their personal history, but also their culture and the history of the group to which they belong". My roots as a clinical psychologist training at the University of East London, on a course renowned as taking a social constructionist approach, have been helpful in developing my understanding of how history might play a key role in thinking about therapeutic approaches in disability services.

Despite Freud's conviction that a degree of intellectual ability is required to undertake analysis (Freud, 1905), O'Driscoll (2009) documents the history of psychoanalytic work for people with intellectual disabilities, showing that suggestions people with intellectual disabilities might benefit from emotional support using a psychoanalytic model in fact date as far back as the 1930s (Clarke, 1933). Hodges (2003) highlights the rise of behavioural models, post-Second World War, and the dominance of behavioural therapy as an approach in services for people with intellectual disabilities at the expense of "talking therapies" over the following decades. Hodges suggests that the acclaimed objectivity that behavioural models assert might also have served to offer professionals and researchers a means of distancing themselves from the emotional impact of working with this population and avoiding the negative feelings stirred up in the face of the pain of disability.

Sinason (1992, 2010) suggested the paucity of access to emotional support for people with disabilities could be someway explained by a societal "death wish" which underlies the marginalisation, exclusion and overlooking of human rights in disability services throughout history. Sinason (2010) has continued to bring attention to society's desire to cut off from uncomfortable feelings about difference and disability. History shows us evidence of how social construction influences policy and how policy dictates treatments of marginalised groups: housing people in out of the way institutions; denying access to education, opportunities and jobs; treating people with contempt; and fundamental breaches of human rights. This concept of a "Death Wish" is further illustrated in a recent documentary *Silenced: The Hidden Story of Disabled Britain* (Scholefield, 2021). Presenter Carrie Burnell exposes the extremes of systemic ableism starting from the "Eugenics movement" and its devastating consequences, causing the annihilation of people with disabilities culminating in forced sterilisation and murder of millions of people with disabilities during the Nazi regime. The realisation of such atrocities led to a departure in scientific interest in eugenics in the UK; however, Burnell highlights the on-going devaluing of people with disabilities and a continued pursuit of correction and perfection aiming to eradicate disability. Human rights remain compromised. Earlier this year Heidi Crowter led a campaign calling for governmental policy change regarding the Abortion Act through the

"Don't Screen Us Out" movement. Crowter was devastated to learn that 90% of women chose to terminate their pregnancy once they learnt their unborn child had Downs Syndrome and she powerfully calls for equal treatment for these unborn babies for whom it remains legal to perform termination of pregnancy up until full term, where for those without known disabilities this would be illegal after 24 weeks. Carter, her partner and her mother sadly lost the tribunal and the Act remains (Topping, 2021). I am reminded of Valerie Sinason's presentation at a conference of a psychotherapy group run by herself and Sheila Hollins; Sinason movingly described the group members talking of their fear and horror of the notion of "amniocentesis", a medical practice aiming to offer expectant parents an opportunity to identify whether or not their infant has a chance of a disability, and subsequently offered counselling to decide whether or not to terminate their pregnancy. Sinason (1999) and Sinason and Hollins (2000) identify this fear of being murdered as an important theme to address in individual therapy with people with intellectual disabilities. I have found that knowledge of medical science and advances in medicine can have differing degrees of impact on the young people and families I have worked with and need to be understood and addressed with care in order to manage the defences that may be functional in protecting against devastating pain.

> In my work with Dawn, a young person with Downs Syndrome, after many sessions drawing flowers and smiling faces she opened up and talked of a trip out to a theatre where she revealed her shock of learning of her diagnosis. She talked about how confusing it was when she saw, in a group of young people with Downs Syndrome that she looked more like these peers than she did her family members. On the other hand, Marcus used his therapy session to act out his and his mum's dream of finding a cure of muscular dystrophy so that other children wouldn't have the same experiences he had. It took time and sensitive attunement to name his feelings and for him to show me that in his heart he knew that any such advances would be too late for him. Another example is Irma, who talked of how she had spent long hours researching possible cures for her son Ismail's intellectual disabilities and autism, raising money to take him for innovative treatments in the USA, only to feel the crushing reality that there was no means of change for him.

Sensitive supervision and support

These painful examples give voice to how difficult it can be to offer talking therapy that gets in touch with this deep level of emotion. In his seminal paper "The unoffered chair", Bender (1993, p. 7) sheds light on how the paucity of therapeutic services available for people with intellectual disabilities may be linked to the fact that "psychotherapy involves intensely relating over quite a long period to another person – a certain kind of intimacy. The giving of this intimacy is more difficult, aversive and more energy consuming when the person is seen as unattractive". Hadley, Greenhill, and Beard (2019, p. 92) suggest that in order to offer therapy to people with intellectual disabilities the therapist needs "to engage in advocacy and be in touch with powerful feelings of exclusion and powerlessness". In its extreme the impact of the work can be so powerful as to traumatise the therapist, as described by Nigel Beail (2015) in his presentation at the IPD conference. Beail illustrated the vicarious trauma that he had experienced and supported in colleagues as a result of bearing witness to the stories of some of the young men that his service offered support to following their experiences of extreme, traumatic abuse. In line with this thinking, it follows that offering therapeutic support for marginalised, stigmatised individuals is challenging work and may not be as attractive as offering therapy to those where change might come more easily. Shouldering the weight of this kind of history, marginalisation and discrimination needs support. Supervision and spaces to voice the pain and powerlessness present in the work, in addition to peer support, are vital elements that help us to provide safe and attuned therapeutic space to individuals with intellectual disabilities and their families. In my own experience, supervision in addition to memberships of a range of groups of interested colleagues (Mental Handicap Workshop, IPD and ID SPIG [a special interest group for the Faculty of Learning Disabilities in the British Psychological Society]) have been immensely important in supporting and maintaining energy and curiosity in my work, and modelling dedication, reflection, and compassion to navigate the work's complexities.

Understanding difference and disability

Understanding the construction of disability and difference can also help to make the important distinction between social, medical, and analytical models of understanding disability and how needs might differ accordingly. Social models of disability propose that it is the environment and context that create profound effects of the individual's impairment and therefore handicap the individual in terms of community participation and choice. Medical models focus on fixing the impairment in order to allow the individual to better access their environment, whilst analytic models focus on the internal experienced of the person with a disability. Wilson (2003) suggests that a relational model can provide bridges between these different models and help the therapist to: a) support individuals in finding ways to engage with society and with the system around them which supports their best potential; b) build confidence and self-esteem; and c) move individuals and their families from a position of powerlessness to power. Brown (2019) also acknowledges the importance of recognising power imbalance in the therapeutic relationship and advocates naming this as a means of supporting meaningful attunement in a relational model of support. This is vital when aiming to work in the UK

National Health Service that is open and free to all and gives voice to the importance of working at different levels within a system. To support individuals within all of these models of disability is key and to work at many different levels of the system it feels as important to demonstrate to commissioning services that consultation, advocacy, and change in the systems supporting individuals is as valuable as face-to-face appointments with individuals offering direct therapeutic intervention.

> *Bobby, Jim, and Suzie lived with their parents in a one-bedroom flat. Bobby had received a diagnosis of Autism Spectrum Condition (ASC) and intellectual disabilities aged six and Jim was also being assessed within the child development service to explore social and communication difficulties. The children had been referred to social care by school with the concern that they were coming to school hungry and unkempt in smelly, dirty clothes. Previous referrals had resulted in Early Help being offered but the family had refused support. A referral was also sent by school to CAMHS asking for individual therapeutic support for Bobby around his behaviour that had deteriorated at home and at school. The family had been previously open to CAMHS and offered behavioural work to support parents to put in clearer boundaries. Sue, Bobby's mum, described how he had a number of sensory issues and seemed to enjoy the sound of smashing glass which resulted in him finding glasses and smashing them on the floor leaving Sue and John worried that the children would be hurt by the broken glass. Our assessment also revealed that the father, John, had recently lost his job and the family were in arrears with their rent and had started using the local food bank. It was clear that the situation was complex and that the stress levels in the whole family system were high and would need multiple levels of support. As a multidisciplinary team we were able to offer work at a number of different levels. We offered consultation to the network to come to a cohesive, shared understanding of the difficulties that the family faced, including analytic thinking about the challenge of parenting a child with a disability and how the parent's confidence might be attacked by their experiences of austerity. This served to co-construct a different narrative for the family and allowed them to accept the help offered by the local authority. By offering supervision to the family support worker, she was able to adapt her parent support model to take account of the neurodevelopmental difficulties that the children faced; the introduction of melatonin supported and brought about improvement in the children's sleep patterns and left everyone in the family better rested. A letter of support to the housing team highlighting how the children's mental health difficulties and disabilities were impacted by their environment and requesting that the housing officer become part of the professional network was also helpful. Finally, working with school and family to better understand Bobby's behaviour and to introduce meaningful activity to support Bobby's narrow interest (i.e., getting a job in the school to undertake the recycling with his TA) also served to foster change in the system which better met Bobby's needs.*

At this point in time, it was clear that individual support for Bobby was not best placed. The family were overwhelmed by their social situation and were not in a position to bring Bobby for regular sessions. We needed to assess the situation and as Anthony Ryle suggests "to push where it moves" or to allow the work to "go where there is readiness and willingness to go" (Potter, 2020, p. 180). I have found it helpful in situations of this kind to draw on both systemic and CAT perspectives and to apply Vygotsky's concept of ZPD (zone of proximal development) to understand how the learning in the system might take place.

Ryle and Kerr (2002, p. 42) noted "the gap between what a child is able to do alone and what he could learn with the provision of appropriate help" and Vygotsky (1978, p. 87) said "what a child does with an adult today she will do in her own tomorrow"; with this ideas in mind, we needed to push the system where it moved and work out the ZPD for the family. In this situation what moved was to re-author the narrative of this family as one with disguised compliance who were reluctant to engage and "hard to help". By understanding their needs and supporting the system to meet those needs in a meaningful way, the family were able to gain confidence and were enabled to access the help they needed.

Balancing support and enabling families

This premise of supporting systems to go it alone can equally be used in supporting families, yet in disability services "going it alone" might be much more complex and needs to be considered carefully. Fletcher (2016) highlights the impact on families of having a child with a disability, explaining that taking in unexpected news and assimilating the uncertain future that inevitably comes with disability can impact the parent's capacity to form a straightforward attachment and interfere with the bonding process between parent and child. Goldberg et al. (1995) suggest that the grief associated with the original diagnosis or loss of the healthy child can be recapitulated with subsequent transitions and when the child's developmental journey veers from a regular or hoped for course. As a consequence, children with disabilities and their families are more likely to encounter difficult times around transitions and are more likely to reach out to services during these difficult times. One key aspect of working within a disabilities service is in supporting the system to understand the lifelong relationship between services and individuals that can challenge the current, politically driven models of access to psychological therapy and short-term work. In our team, we have aimed to understand the complexities that accompany long relationships between service user and service by naming and developing awareness of the wavering line between dependency and enabling. The helping relationship can be challenged in service where the difficulties don't go away and increasing referrals and long waiting lists can leave staff feeling overwhelmed and pressured to meet goals and complete work in a short period of time. I have drawn on my experience of working using systemic models to help address these dilemmas. By advocating and supporting peer support and through offering regular reviews, we have aimed to offer services that work alongside families to co-create different narratives within family life and to support young people and parents to speak up within their wider systems, school, medical, and social services. Some examples of this kind of work are offering different sorts of groups to families and young people, where there is an element of meeting others and learning from one another's experiences alongside psychoeducation and expert support. Working along the lines of "episodes of care" has helped us to begin to maintain boundaries to our work and to offer enabling support.

> Mary, a young psychologist was working with Mark's mum, Sammy. She (Mary) felt that the work was going well and they had met their intended goals with the work. However, every time Mary talked about the prospect of finishing their work, Sammy would bring a new issue of concern. There is no doubt that these issues brought up were real and causing Sammy and her son Mark great difficulty, but we have tried to understand this common experience in our service using the premise of dependency (Sinason and Hollins, 2000) and enabling. Mary brought her work with Sammy to her supervision to explore this experience and we agreed that developing a narrative with Sammy which described the work as an "episode of care" might meet the family's needs, alongside our need to meet the demands of a long waiting list and high numbers of new referrals. We were conscious that we did not want Sammy to feel abandoned or rejected which might mirror her more negative experience of service but thought if we could offer arm's length support when goals had been met, this might serve as a safety net that increased Sammy's confidence that she could re-enter the service when needed in future. We consulted with a group of parents in the service and developed a parent-facilitated group for those who have used our services but who didn't feel quite ready to go it alone. The aim of this group is to foster a long-term relationship with the service rather than particular members of the team in an enabling way. Research with adolescents does show that children and families are happier to engage with people they know but a high staff turnover, particularly in the current NHS, often means people were returning to a new therapist. Our aim is to try to embody the identity of the work in the service as well as the individuals.

Building confidence

Building confidence is without doubt one of the most key issues in working with disability. During my career I have had the privilege of working closely with Professor Maria Rhode both as a newly qualified clinical psychologist and in my current role and have continued to gain from her insights. Professor Rhode has undertaken a research project in our disability CAMHS service which we were pleased to support; it included an intensive psychotherapeutic approach with parents and siblings of children where a diagnosis of autism has been given or is suspected and sought to explore the impact of an intensive relational approach in improving outcomes around developing confidence in parents. Building on the work of Professor Green and colleagues in Manchester (Green and Dunn, 2008; Green et al., 2008) and Daniel Stern (1985, 1990, 1998) and thinking about early detections of vulnerabilities to diagnosis, Rhode coined the term "cycles of discouragement" (Rhode and Grayson, 2021, n.p.). Rhode noticed that the overwhelming nature of gaze in infants genetically vulnerable to neuro-diverse or atypical brain development, can have a profound effect on the adoring parental gaze from the earliest days of bonding. This has been a most helpful means of understanding issues from both the child and the parent's perspective. Winnicott (1965) noted that our first understanding of ourselves is reflected in the eyes of those who first see us. Fletcher (2016), among others, has written eloquently of the experience of parents from an attachment perspective and suggested that bonding can be interrupted by the stresses resulting from the birth of a child with disabilities. Rhode (2021) proposes the importance of the therapist being able to "model receptivity", "to empower the parents and support their capacity to observe" (n.p.), and to convey a strong sense that the behaviour is meaningful and is a powerful communication tool where typical communication means may be limited or compromised by the functional disabilities.

Rhode states that the significant features of intervention adhering to this understanding will include parental involvement central to agreeing therapeutic support, empathy with the family's emotional experience, focus on meaning, parental support, and the promotion of receptive behaviour. By improving observational skills and understanding in the parents, the workers can support a

> virtuous circle of mutual encouragement between parent and child instead of the vicious circle of discouragement between parents and child in which repeated experiences of invalidation lead the parents to expect nothing else and not to notice the often faint indications that the child might be more open to contact
>
> (Rhode and Grayson, 2021, n.p.).

This focus on a cycle of encouragement has been key in our work for many different models in our service and we have found it is a powerful and necessary adjunct to the transitional positive behavioural models that dominate in disabilities services today. The cycle of encouragement, evident in work with David and his family (discussed below), offers an illustration of how this concept has been a key tenet of thinking about disability and how disability might impact on parental confidence.

David came to our service at the suggestion of his school Special Educational Needs Co-ordinator (SENCO) who had noticed an increasing reluctance to go to his lessons and a high number of unauthorised absences at school. David was eight years old with an already long history of struggling to engage with school. There had been referrals to our service in the past but family had been reluctant to engage in work after assessment and had turned down offers of support. In our assessment session his parents described how he was spending more and more time in his bedroom and was reluctant to engage with his parents or his younger siblings other than with angry outbursts. The assessment also uncovered that David was engaging in long complex rituals before school which, at times, would leave him unable to attend as he was worried about not attending on time. David's parents were working hard to encourage him but their own anxiety about potential tantrums was clear in our first session. It became clear that since David was a small child his anxiety had left the family feeling hopeless and helpless and they had increasingly moulded their lives around adhering to David's rituals and narrow interests; for instance, Janis, David's mum told us about how when he was three, she and David were regularly out in the rain watching the water swirl into the drains for many hours at a time. We talked about David's early experience and it was clear that his story was saturated with anxiety. The pregnancy had been difficult with much of the third trimester having David's mum in hospital, away from her older children, and lying flat (as there were complications that left them fearing a late miscarriage). The birth was complicated with a long hard labour that resulted in a "Ventouse delivery". The early days were also difficult with Janis struggling to juggle her scratchy new baby who wanted to feed all the time with the older siblings whom she felt she had neglected whilst being in hospital. The couple talked about the stress levels being high, little family support, and additional pressures at work for Fred (dad) as he tried to be supportive to Janis and felt he was cutting corners at work to make time for the family. Janis revealed that she had felt David was controlling her from before he was born and the only way she could manage was to give into his demands, first to be fed, later to watch water going down the drains, and many other little rituals. Fred said he shut out from the dyad of David and Janis and the other two children appeared to be getting on with things so he felt useless and distressed. Following our assessment, we formulated a cycle of discouragement and saw that this had been exacerbated in the past by contact with the service where parent support had been offered leaving the parents feeling blamed and unheard. We let them know we were not surprised that they were exhausted and felt this way and praised them for their tenacity and their strength with supporting David to meet his needs. With slow and careful work, adhering to Rhode's principles, we were able to build up rapport and consequently to build up confidence. David was supported by his parents to attend school and his parents were encouraged to engage extended family support so that they could attend to their older children and to themselves, giving them a different perspective and beginning to develop cycles of encouragement together.

Attending to the feelings of blame and critical voice

In my clinical experience it is common for parents to hear criticism when we ask them about difficulties with behaviour. Parents report the experience of often having had to fight for their child's needs to be understood at every stage of their life. In addition, when the dominant narrative in UK society is the likes of "Super Nanny", "Britain's Best Parent", and endless expertise on social media platforms and you have a child who is not fitting with the social norms, it is not surprising that there can be a propensity to hear "experts" as critical. Such ubiquitous narratives of perfect parenting may exacerbate the feelings linked to the challenges of parenting a child with additional needs and further lead to feelings of being inadequate or judged. On top of that, attending services where they are asked to talk about and reflect on their own part in the child's perceived difficulties may be experienced as a further judgement of parenting capacity. It is vital therefore to build a trusting space and a rapport with families. In a political landscape where mental health needs are increasingly being seen as being ameliorated by a limited number of sessions, this capacity for building relationship can be overlooked. As a team, we have tried to develop means of gently and carefully addressing this issue as early in the work as possible by drawing on our understanding of attachment, containment, neuropsychology, and relational intelligence.

In the majority of therapeutic models, the early relationship between infant and carer is examined to give the theoretical foundations. An understanding of this initial attachment can give great insight in to a young person's current difficulties. In psychoanalytic models (Psychoanalytic psychotherapy or cognitive analytic therapy) these early relationships are understood to give a blueprint for later relationships and there are some areas that I have found particularly relevant in helping developing understanding of relationships for people with disabilities with their families. Music (2011) gives a comprehensive account of the interplay between attachment relationships and neuropsychological development. He revisits some of the original attachment research (a child goes to hospital) and the extensive and terribly distressing clinical material that transpired as a result of the discovery of Romanian orphanages where severe neglect has shown the impact on actual brain development (Chugani et al., 2001). Music (2011, p. 93) further investigates the impact of trauma on brain development, giving a convincing explanation of how "experience affects the brain, particularly very bad experiences such as of severe trauma or neglect".

Music (2011) explores the interactions between brain development and emotional responses. In a slightly earlier work, Siegel (2007) shows how those with psychological or psychiatric issues show fewer interconnections between areas of the brain than those with fewer issues. Music (2009) then used this phenomenon to help understand different emotional responses in the therapy room. We also use this as a means of supporting parents and young people to further understand their emotional responses and how to respond to the child's anxiety.

Bion (1962) shows how his concept of containment is fundamental to developing thinking as by containing and processing a child's primal emotional responses the carer can demonstrate how thinking is possible and how to do it. Hodges (2003) describes how helpful this concept is in working with children and families where disability is present. Douglas (2007) also shows how containment and reciprocity are vital in developing attunement that supports developing relationships, social communication, and emotional regulation and concludes that knowledge of these techniques is an asset in working with children for whom such concepts are difficult to grasp.

Many authors have understood that the birth of a child with disabilities can lead to the need to process the loss of the expected child and this process may have vastly different degrees of emotional impact ranging from adjustment to trauma (Hodges, 2003; Ditchfield, 1992; Fletcher, 2016; Beaumont, 2016; Bicknell, 1983). The concept of containment has therefore also become a bedrock to our team's efforts in working with children and families with disabilities; it is relevant with individual, parent work, supervision, and consultation or support for other agencies:

> In our work with Fiona's network we aimed to understand Fiona's extremely difficult behaviour in the context of her history of abuse; the staff struggled to understand why she would keep getting into trouble, escaping from her residential unit, and felt forced into placing more and more restrictions to manage the risk. By exploring her history, we were able to support the team to understand that the behaviour and the consequences were mirroring her experience of abuse; when she felt anxious the system was asserting control, increasing her anxiety and leaving her with the only response to flee. The team began to build up activities that supported Fiona and contained her anxiety when it flared, rather than asserting control. They found relationships improved and she was more able to talk about her anxiety. Containing the anxiety of the team helped them to contain Fiona's anxiety and her behaviour began to diminish.

In more recent years I have undertaken training in cognitive analytic therapy. An interest that was first sparked by the links between ACAT (Association of Cognitive Analytic Therapists) and the IPD (Institute of Psychotherapy and Disability). In cognitive analytic therapy we understand that early experiences can form a blueprint for later relationships through the formation of reciprocal roles: if we experience neglectful care as a child, we might see that a reciprocal role develops where as an adult we resentfully care for others and for ourselves. Jenaway (2007) has explored attachment and the development of reciprocal roles through a CAT lens and applied a developmental model of reciprocal roles and the parents' role to help the baby develop a middle ground of loving but with boundaries and limits to achieve good enough care. Many authors have noted that children with learning disabilities are frequently less responsive to their caregivers and do not initiate interactions. Similarly, their signals may be harder to interpret which might result in complex attachments developing between carer and child. As a result, we have wondered if parents may fear they have caused the disability (blaming – blamed) which is a further threat to secure attachment. The parents' own attachment patterns and reciprocal roles will also input on their capacity to manage the child's feelings to reaching a middle ground. Another reciprocal role that we have identified is a "grieving to giving grief" supporting network.

Ahmadi (2019) also notes how useful the concept of reformulation can be in working with families affected by trauma, disadvantage, and austerity, as it can support recognition that the difficulties they are beyond their control. Ahmadi (2019, p. 82) explains: "being able to conceptualise their experience, validated in therapy, can be empowering by reducing self-blame and self-recrimination which otherwise would exacerbate reciprocal role procedures that are damaging to themselves and to their children".

Varela and Franks (2018) note that if we are able to recognise that when our expertise or need to be in a position of power or knowledge is challenged within our therapeutic roles, or in supporting parents and colleagues, and can acknowledge the distress this might cause us, we are more likely to be able to attune to our feelings and respond in a helpful way, rather than fall into a reciprocal role procedure which might further entrench the challenges faced.

I have found that an understanding of these concepts can similarly be a powerful tool in supporting families to recognise and respond to the experience of disability in their family, for which blame and a search for causes can become destructive to both them and to their children.

Our work with Omid and Greta, parents of Maya – an eight-year-old girl with a diagnosis of social communication difficulties, significant language delay, and moderate learning disabilities – gives an illustration of how important attending to these issues can be in maintaining a supportive, helpful position. Greta and Omid had worked with the team when Maya was three and had received the diagnosis within the child development part of our service. They had diligently engaged in the post diagnostic support and Maya had started mainstream school with support. She initially did well and the CDT closed the case, however, as she got older the gap between her abilities and the abilities of her peers became more and more stark. Omid was devastated and contacted the service filled with rage, feeling that the services had let them down. In reopening Maya's case we found that Greta too was feeling devastated but had begun to withdraw from previously supportive relationships as she found even the most innocuous comments of her friends increasingly painful. Following every contact, we received an angry email fearing that access to services was being withheld or criticising the skills and knowledge base of the therapists offering support, stressing that the services offered were not sufficient. Maya's behaviour at home and at school had started to deteriorate and she was regularly found to be screaming in the face of any demand placed on her, from putting her shoes on to getting ready for bed. Colleagues in social care had similar experience with duty calls pleading for additional support and highly critical responses to the carers that were provided. Staff were becoming disheartened, offended, and worried that they were starting to feel they might respond in an unprofessional manner. We arranged a professionals meeting with an external facilitator and in using a mentalising, thinking-together model (AMBIT – Adaptive Mentalisation Based Integrative Treatment [Bevington et al., 2017]) we were able to explore the "giving (us) grief" position and understand the family's responses in terms of "fight flight freeze" deep set anxiety and fear in the realisation that Maya would not be getting better but that her future might present the family with more and more challenges. The realisation of the extent of Maya's difficulties and seeing how far this departed from her expected or hoped for development seemed to be underpinning the parent's response. In addition, our sessions were revealing different experiences in the parents' own attachment patterns that left them with few resources to steel themselves for the challenges they faced. Omid had lost his mother at an early age and Greta had suffered from extreme anxiety and been horribly bullied at school. We were able to support the network to understand that the parents' experience of engaging with helping services had stirred up feelings linked to these early experiences. The parents were faced with a vicious circle of either feeling overwhelmed and angry or projecting their support network from this anger by withdrawing from support. This dilemma, in turn, left the network with strong feelings about the family, experiencing them as overwhelming and responding to the overwhelm by putting in boundaries and restricting the forms of communication (i.e., not responding to angry emails). The network's response unwittingly left Omid and Greta feeling overlooked, neglected, and alone, mirroring the feelings they had as a result of their early experiences and further compounding their angry, hopeless, and helpless responses.

Conclusion

As a Clinical Psychologist I have drawn on many different models to inform my work and been influenced by many different authors and mentors. I have highlighted what I believe to be the key tenets of working in disability services. By treating people with respect and understanding how history, culture, and societies' construction of difficulties can impact on individuals, their families, and support networks, we can offer support that is effective in bringing about change, however small. By identifying and attending to the experiences of disability and difference, the internal critical voice, and painful feelings of blame and shame we can support individuals and families to build confidence and feel enabled towards independence. In addition, mobilising support through supervision and linking with thoughtful, reflective colleagues seems vital in maintaining curiosity, compassion and dedication in our work. In my search for eclecticism, I hope to have given an illustration of how, understanding and bringing models together, we can work together as a cohesive multidisciplinary team to support children and families with disabilities effectively and to allow us to offer a chair for emotional support to those people with intellectual disabilities who are so commonly overlooked and marginalised.

Bibliography

Ahmadi, J.F.D., (2019). The intergenerational transmission of the adverse effects of inequality. In Lloyd, J. and Pollard. R., *Cognitive Analytic Therapy and the Politics of Mental Health*, 77–91. London, New York: Routledge.

Baum, S. and Lynggaard, H. (2006). (Eds). *Intellectual Disabilities: A Systemic Approach*. London, New York: Karnac.

Beail, N. (2015), *Presentation 2nd Oct 2015: "Vicarious Trauma in therapy"*. IPD Annual Conference, AGM and workshop – "Working together: Psychotherapy and Positive Behaviour Support".

Beaumont, H. (2016). *Hole in the Heart: Bringing Up Beth*. Brighton: Myriad.

Bender, M. (1993). The unoffered chair: the history of therapeutic distain towards people with learning disabilities. *Clinical Psychology Forum*, 43, 2–6.

Bevington, D., Fuggle, P., Cracknell. L and Fonagy, P. (2017). *Adaptive Mentalisation-Based Integrative Treatment: A Guide for Teams to Develop Systems of Care*. Oxford:Oxford University Press.

Bicknell, J. (1983). The Psychopathology of Handicap. *British Journal of Medical Psychology*, 56(2), 167–178.

Bion, W. (1962). *A Theory of Thinking in Second Thoughts*. London: Karnac.

Britain Best Parents? (2020). Channel 4.

Brown, H. (2019). Reciprocal Roles in an Unequal World. In Lloyd, J. and Pollard, R. *Cognitive Analytic Therapy and the Politics of Mental Health*. London, New York: Routledge, 20–37.

Chinn, D. and Abraham, E. (2016). Using 'candidacy' as a framework for understanding access to mainstream psychological treatment for people with intellectual disabilities and common mental health problems within the English Improving Access to Psychological Therapies service. *Journal of Intellectual Disability Research*, 60(6), Jun, 571–582.

Chugani, H.T., Behen, M.E.Muzik, O., Juhasz, C. Nagy, F. and Chugani, D.C. (2001). Local Brain functional activity following early deprivation: a study of post-institutionaliszed Romanian Orphans. *Neuroimage*, 14(6), 1290–1301.

Clarke, P. (1933). *The Nature and Treatment of Amentia*. Paris:Bailliere.

Cooper, S.A.Smiley, E., Morrison, J., Williamson, A. and Allan, L. (2007) Mental Illness in adults with Intellectual Disabilities: Prevalence and associated factors. *The British Journal of Psychiatry, 190*, 27–35.

Corbett., A. (2019). *Intellectual Disabilities and Psychotherapy*. London: Routledge.

Department of Health. (2001). *Valuing People: A New Strategy for Learning Disability for the 21st Century*. London: Department of Health.

Department of Health. (2009). *Valuing People Now. A New Three-Year Strategy for People with Learning Disabilities*. London: Department of Health.

Department of Health. (2010). *Equalities Act*. London: Department of Health.

Department of Health. (2012). *Transforming Care: A national response to Winterbourne View Hospital*. London: Department of Health.

Disabilities Rights Commission. (2006). *Equal Treatment: Closing the Gap*. Stratford-upon Avon: Disability Rights Commission.

Ditchfield, H. (1992). The birth of a child with a mental handicap: coping with loss. In A. Waitman and S. Conboy-Hill (eds.), *Psychotherapy and Mental Handicap*, 9–23. London: Sage.

Douglas, H. (2007). *Containment and Reciprocity: Integrating Psychoanalytic Theory and Child Development Research for Work with Children*. London, New York: Routledge.

Emerson, E. and Hatton, C. (2007). Mental Health of Children and Adolescents with Intellectual Disabilities in Britain. *The British Journal of Psychiatry*, 191(6), 493–499.

Fletcher, H. K. (2016). Attachment relationships between parents and their children: the impact of the loss of the healthy child. In Fletcher H.K., Flood, A. and Hare, D.J. (eds), *Attachment in Intellectual and Developmental Disability: A Clinician's Guide to Practice and Research*. Chichester: Wiley.

Freud, S. (1905). Fragment of an Analysis of a Case of Hysteria. *The Standard Edition of the Complete Psychological Works of Sigmund Freud, Volume VII (1901–1905): A Case of Hysteria, Three Essays on Sexuality and Other Works*, 3–122. London: The Hogarth Press.

Goldberg, D., Magill, L.Hale, J.Damaskinidou, K., Paul, J. and Tham, S. (1995). *Protection and loss: working with learning disabled adults and their families. Journal of Family Therapy*, 17, 263–280.

Green, J. and G. Dunn. (2008). Using intervention trials in developmental psychiatry to illuminate basic science. *British Journal of Psychiatry*, 192(5), 323–325.

Green, J., M.W. Wan, and M. Deklyen, (2008). *Attachment insecurity and attachment disorder*. In P. Tyrer and K.R. Silk (eds.), *Cambridge Textbook of Effective Treatments in Psychiatry*, 748–755. Cambridge: Cambridge University Press.

Hadley, E, Greenhill, B., and Beard, K. (2019). Using CAT to bridge the gap: attending to the ultimate and the intimate. In Lloyd, J. and Pollard. R. (eds.), *Cognitive Analytic Therapy and the Politics of Mental Health*, 92–111. London, New York: Routledge.

Hodges, S. (2003). *Counselling Adults with Learning Disabilities*. New York: Palgrave Macmillan.

Jenaway, A., (2007). Using Cognitive Analytic Therapy with parents: some theory and a case report. *Reformulation*, Winter, 12–15.

Mencap. (2004). *Treat Me Right!* London: Mencap.

Mencap. (2007). *Death by Indifference*. London: Mencap.

Michaels, J. (2008). *Health for All: Report of the Independent Enquiry into Access to Healthcare for People with Learning Disabilities*. London: Department of Health.

Music, G. (2009). Neuroscience and Child Psychotherapy. In M. Lanyado and A. Horne (eds.), *The Handbook of Child and Adolescent Psychotherapy* (2nd Edition). London: Routledge.

Music, G. (2011). *Nurturing Natures: Attachment and Children's Emotional, Sociocultural and Brain Development*. Hove and New York: Psychology Press.

NOT SPECIAL NEEDS – World Down Syndrome Day #NotSpecialNeeds. CoorDown. https://www.youtube.com/watch?v=kNMJaXuFuWQ. 16 March 2017. YouTube.

O'Driscoll, D. (2009). Psychotherapy and intellectual disability: a historical view. In T. Cottis (ed.), *Intellectual Disability, Trauma and Psychotherapy*, 9–28. Hove: Routledge.

Potter, S. (2020). *Therapy as a Map: A Cognitive Analytic Approach to Helping Relationships*. Shoreham-by-Sea: Pavilion Publishing.

Potter, S. (2014). The Helper's Dance List. In Lloyd, J. and Clayton, P. (eds.), *Cognitive Analytic Therapy for People with Intellectual Disabilities and their Carers*, 89–97. London, Philadelphia: Jessica Kingsley.

Rhode, M. and Grayson, K. (2021). An Observationally and Psychoanalytically Informed Parent-Toddler Intervention for Young Children at Risk of ASD: An Audited Case Series and Convergences with Organicist Approaches. In Fitzgerald, M. (ed.), *Autism Spectrum Disorder, Heterogeneity, Neurobiology and Intervention*. London: IntechOpen.

Ryle, A. and Kerr, I. (2002). *Introducing Cognitive Analytic Therapy: Principles and Practice*. Chichester: Wiley.

Siegel, D.J. (2007). *The Mindful Brain: Reflection and Attunement in the Cultivation of Well-Being*. New York: Norton.

Scholefield, K. (dir.). (2021). *Silenced: The Hidden Story of Disability in Britain*. BBC, 9th January.

Sinason, V. (1992). *Mental Handicap and the Human Condition: New Approaches from the Tavistock*. London: Free Association Press.

Sinason, V. and Stokes, J. (1992). Secondary Handicap as a defence. In A. Waitman and S. Conboy-Hill (eds.), *Psychotherapy and Mental Handicap*, 45–58. London: Sage.

Sinason, V. (1999). The psychotherapeutic needs of the learning disabled and multiply disabled child. In M. Lanyado and A. Horne (eds.), *The Handbook of Child and Adolescent Psychotherapy*, 415–427. London: Routledge.

Sinason, V. (2010). *Mental Handicap and the Human Condition: An Analytic Approach to Intellectual Disability*. London: Free Association Press.

Sinason, V., and Hollins, S. (2000). Psychotherapy, learning disabilities and trauma, new perspectives. *British Journal of Psychiatry*, 176, 32–36.

Stern, D., (1985). *The Interpersonal World of the Infant: A View from Psychoanalysis and Developmental Psychology*. New York: Basic Books.

Stern, D. (1990). Joy and satisfaction in infancy. In R. Glick and S. Bone. (eds.), *Pleasure Beyond the Pleasure Principal*. New Haven, CT: Yale University Press.

Stern, D. (1998). *Diary of a Baby*. New York: Basic Books.

Supernanny. (2004–2011). Channel 4.

Symington, N. (1992). Countertransference with mentally handicapped clients. In A. Waitman and S. Conboy-Hill (eds.), *Psychotherapy and Mental Handicap*, 132–138. London: Sage.

Topping, A. (2021). Woman with Down's syndrome loses UK abortion law case. *The Guardian*, 23rd September.

Varela, J. and Franks, L. (2018). Responding not reacting to challenging behaviour a reformulation approach. In Lloyd, J. and Pollard, R. (eds.), *Cognitive Analytic Therapy and the Politics of Mental Health*, 129–143. London, New York. Routledge.

Vygotsky, L.S. (1978). *Mind in Society: The Development of Higher Psychological Processes*. Cambridge, MA: Harvard University Press.

Whittle, K. L., Fisher, R.W., Peppermund, S., and Troller, J. (2019). Access to mental health services: The experiences of people with intellectual disabilities. *Journal of Applied Research in Intellectual Disabilities*, 32(2), 368–379.

Wilson, S. (2003). *Disability, Counselling and Psychotherapy: Challenges and Opportunities*. New York: Palgrave Macmillan.

Winnicott, D. (1965). *The Maturational Processes and the Facilitating Environment*. London: Hogarth Press

Chapter 12

Treating Psychosis with Respect
Including the Contribution of Dr Phoebe Caldwell

Elspeth Bradley

This is the chapter I wish I could have had early on in my work as a psychiatrist / psychotherapist. The chapter embraces those with different sensory worlds – deafblindness, autism – as well as touching on concepts of attachment, trauma and interoception, exploring the relevance of these in the experience of our cohesive sense of self and in turn the relevance of this in mental distress and behaviours that challenge. Here I try to give space to the perspective of the other – to the extent we can ever understand the world of another, especially those whose sensory and lived experiences are outside of our own.

I am also trying to draw attention to "we are all us" – just different experiences of the world – and to give voice to the perspective of the less empowered, rather than that of the therapist. So, the sentiment of these last few lines just written is what I would like to share:

I am informed by Intensive Interaction approaches and the work of Phoebe Caldwell (2007; 2018a), an Intensive Interaction therapist, who has kindly contributed to this chapter several vignettes to illustrate this approach.

Intensive Interaction uses body language, to engage emotionally with people with intellectual disabilities (IDD), autism (ASD) and others (see later), particularly those with profound communication and cognitive disabilities, some of whom historically have been described as "locked in their own world", "egocentric" or even "psychotic". Intensive Interaction focuses on relationships between people rather than on symptoms and behaviours. Humans are relational beings; without relationships our very survival is in peril, such as is the case for the human infant who, without meaningful relationships, does not thrive (Spitz, 1945). Relationships are not possible without communication. Babies are born with capacities to communicate (e.g., crying, smiling and imitating) and an instinctive desire for companionship (Zeedyk, 2008, n.d.; Trevarthen and Delafield-Butt, 2017). Children and adults with communication difficulties – born into a world where their communicative attempts are not understood or ignored – are at risk of isolation, loneliness, developmental handicaps, bullying, mental and physical ill health, as well as misdiagnoses of the impact on health of these lived experiences.

DOI: 10.4324/9781003646242-16

The concept of using a person's personal body language, as a means of communicating purposively with individuals with communication difficulties and developmental disabilities was first introduced by Ephraim who named it "augmented mothering" (Ephraim, 1990), later to be renamed Intensive Interaction (Nind and Hewett, 1994). The approach has subsequently been informed by developmental and intersubjectivity theorists and clinicians such as Beebe (Beebe and Lachmann, 1988; Beebe, Lachmann and Jaffe, 1997; Beebe, 2014), Bruner (Bruner, 2014), Stern (Stern, 1985), Trevarthen (Trevarthen, 2013, 2014, 2016; Trevarthen and Delafield-Butt, 2017) and Zeedyk (Zeedyk, 2008) as well as Intensive Interaction practitioners (e.g., Caldwell, 2008; Caldwell et al., 2019). While behavioural interventions focus on behaviours themselves and aim to change those behaviours deemed to be socially undesirable or non-adaptive, in Intensive Interaction the focus is on those behaviours that have meaning for the individual and valuing these as significant to that person (Davies et al., 2008, p. 87).

Trevarthen describes the communicating partner entering into a collaboration with the "*intentions*" of the other, "assisting [them] to a higher level of skill, motivation or emotional regulation" (Trevarthen, 2008, p. 33).

It is about an exchange, sharing and respect, about learning from each other and learning to value what is important to our communicating partner – and so showing them how valuable they are, giving them a sense of their intrinsic worth as people (Caldwell, 2008, p. 183). Below, brief vignettes of this way of working have been kindly provided by Dr Phoebe Caldwell.

First vignette provided by Dr Phoebe Caldwell:

Finding a way to communicate with Gabriel (Caldwell, 2018a, 2018b)

Gabriel has no speech and when I was asked to see him, the psychologist told me, "If you can work with Gabriel, you can work with anyone". And it did seem difficult. He had no interest at all in people, but paced round the room. He pushed me aside (without aggression) but as if I were a lump of furniture. Eventually he picked up a rubber glove and sat on the floor, flicking his left hand with the glove. I sat beside him with another glove; I am following his body language, I am looking at not only at what he is doing, but rather more importantly, how he is doing it, since the manner of his initiatives is a window on how he is feeling. Every time he moved, I responded with a similar rhythm on my own hand. After a while he began to flick his wrist and glance up to see if I would respond. I then tried tapping the rhythm on his knee but he got up and left. His support worker said, "his allowing me to sit with him was a plus, since normally if one tried to engage his attention, he would start to self-injure". After a pause, Gabriel started flicking in the same way with string, so I picked up a length and resumed sitting by him, answering to his initiatives.

He gradually became more interested in what I was doing, to the point where he would shake the string and then look round deliberately to see if I would respond in kind. By now he was looking directly at me and starting to smile. He put a bead on his string and when I added one to mine, his smile deepened and he began to look round the room to see if anyone else was interested. After lunch he came back and picked up a balloon and half inflated it – and released it so that the air streamed into his ear.

By now Gabriel knew that if he made an initiative, I would respond. He introduced different activities to test this. Walking over to the sink, he banged it and looked round to see if I would do the same. Since I had witnessed his letting the balloon deflate into his ear, I knew that this was a signal he recognised, so I blew in his ear and then banged the sink. He turned back and, close up, looked deeply into my eyes; he was totally engaged and glowing with pleasure. It was a most intimate moment.

> People will say I have known this person for years but I have never really known them ... then suddenly ... we are in complete equality ... we talk a lot about equality and valuing people but real equality is when you use the same language with each other, the same emotional language ... and you value each other.
>
> (Caldwell, 2007, n. p.)

This extraordinary "moment of meeting" with Gabriel (Davis, 2015; Stern, 1985) shown on video and articulated by Phoebe comes at the end of two days working with Gabriel, an individual with learning (intellectual and developmental) disability (IDD) and autism (ASD) (American Psychiatric Association, 2013) who spends his waking hours avoiding others and in seemingly purposeless behaviours such as running back and forth, twiddling pieces of string, and banging his head against hard surfaces. Gabriel, who is non-verbal and usually gives no eye contact, is seen looking intently at Dr Caldwell's face; his palpable curiosity and interest in her evoke a felt sense of mutual trust and vulnerability. What has happened? How has this meaningful engagement with Gabriel been possible after a lifetime of him ignoring and avoiding people? Can an understanding of this encounter inform our treating psychosis with respect?

Tuning into Gabriel (Caldwell, 2018b)

Autistic people have difficulty processing incoming sensory information and the brain is easily sensorily overloaded. The approach I was using is one that I had learned from Geraint Ephraim, Clinical Psychologist at Harperbury Hospital. Called "Intensive Interaction", this technique involves using an individual's personal body language to communicate, not just by copying what they are doing but by responding to how they are doing it, which allows one to tune into their affective state. The rationale is that the skilled partner is using signals that are easy to process. In a world where their sensory processing is scrambled, these have immediate meaning. They provide recognisable markers to which they can refer.

One of the problems faced by people who support autistic individuals is that we assume that they are experiencing the same sensory intake as we do. So, we base our strategies and make behavioural judgements based on what happens to us, rather than taking into account their sensory hyper- and hypo-sensitivities and other sensory deficits. In trying to frog-march them into a world that the brain cannot process, we increase their stress and anxiety, with behavioural consequences. Many complain of a loss of sense of self.

True respect places us alongside the individual by taking the trouble to learn their emotional language. Anxiety is reduced when we communicate within the parameters of intimate attention (Caldwell, 2018b, 2018c).

This deeper understanding of the importance of Intensive Interaction as an authentic and profound opportunity for equal relationship in the moment between two people resonates with the "I-Thou" way of engaging with the world (Buber and Kaufmann, 1970). The need for the therapist to immerse themselves in the subjective experience of the patient as a way to more fully understand developmental needs and emerging affect, is also recognised in more traditional "talking" therapies (Kohut, Goldberg and Stepansky, 1984).

Examples of Intensive Interaction approaches in practice:

Orphans in Romania

Davies et al. (2008) studied the use of Intensive Interaction in a sample of Romanian children classified as "irrecuperable", with many having suffered a triple handicap: born with a mental or physical handicap, being abandoned by parents and having experienced a lifetime of chronic neglect in state care thereafter (Davies et al., 2008, p. 85). Young volunteers were trained in the basic approach of Intensive Interaction so that they could incorporate this into their ways of working with these children. Quantitative and qualitative measurements and analyses were conducted. The use of imitative responses was found to have a significant impact on the children's eye gaze to their volunteer partners. All volunteers reported positive changes in their engagement with the children under their care, including increase in child attention to them, increased positive affect displayed by the child, increased proximity to others, and increased flexibility and ease in interactions; the latter permitted spontaneous creation of new games and routines.

Individuals with congenital deafblindness

With individuals who have congenital deafblindness (deafblind), the communicating partner has to very deliberately step outside his reality of a visual landscape to embrace a tactile landscape. "It is the responsibility of the communication partner to think themselves into the perceptual world of the deafblind person and to participate in joint activities from that person's perspective" (Hart, 2008, p. 67). Here joint attention has to be to the same external object in a tactile manner. This joint attention in the same sensory landscape is the shared social reality from which shared practical and emotional communication can develop. Hart comments: "In order to talk about events in the past [or the future] it is first necessary to share communicative landscapes fully in the present" (Hart, 2008, p. 79).

Intensive Interaction and dementia (Adaptive Interaction)

In dementia the combination of diminishing cognitive and functional capacities, personal response to these losses, as well as family, friends and colleague's responses to the adult they are no longer able to engage in conversation, conspires to disengage the adult with dementia from their network of current and past relationships and instead they retreat into their own world. Loneliness, anxiety, fear and psychotic symptoms such as hallucinations and paranoid delusions (some of which may be misinterpretations associated with failing sensory reception) are frequently described (Brendel and Stern, 2005). Some with dementia exhibit persistent body movements involving stimulation of their own bodies such as rubbing their legs, chewing their fingers and pulling at items of their clothing (Ellis and Astell, 2018). These self-stimulatory, repetitive behaviours have been described as perhaps representing "a last desperate bid to remain psychologically alive" (Kitwood, 1997, p. 16). As they also seem to be ones that the person recognises (Ellis and Astell, 2018 and below), is it possible these behaviours might be used as a basis of communication between the adult with dementia and their care providers, thus maintaining emotional engagement with others so that the individual might continue to be anchored in the world outside of themselves, thus staving off loneliness and anxiety?

Second vignette provided by Dr Phoebe Caldwell:

> A member of my family, in the last stages of dementia, is scratching her sheet. She no longer recognises me. When I scratch back the same rhythm, her posture alters, her head tilts towards me and she is alert for a short while. It is the last time we really meet each other.
>
> (P. Caldwell, personal communication, 2018)

Ellis and Astell (2018) explore an Intensive Interaction approach in the support of individuals with dementia where speech-based activities are no longer meaningful. They found that patients had retained a varied set of early communication behaviours including eye gaze, movements and sounds, coupled with a desire to interact with other people. They further observed that care providers in dementia understandably come with the perspective of someone with a full range of speech and may see "proper" communication between people as the exchange of messages. In this context the sounds of the person with dementia for example are not considered as a form of communication but rather a symptom of dementia and indeed may come to be seen as problem behaviour. As dementia progresses the individual experiences diminishing capacities and changes in their sensory and perceptual realities (landscape); similar to the initially different landscapes of the deafblind and typically sighted partner, when one partner has progressive dementia, in order to understand each other, common ground (a shared reality) has to be found. In their research on Intensive Interaction with individuals with dementia, Ellis and Astell have developed detailed process charts to assist care providers communicate without words (Ellis and Astell, 2018, pp. 172–176). They describe an important difference (in working with adults with dementia using the Intensive Interaction approach) is in recognising that memory problems, typical in this population, mean that the individual may not remember previous interactions (although a memory of the rhythm in these interactions may still remain). Hence the communicating partner has to come prepared that interactions may start anew each time of meeting; the communicating partner has to adapt to whichever communicative behaviours the person is engaging in at any particular time. For this reason, they name their approach *Adaptive Interaction.*

Information sought to inform Adaptive Interaction includes:

1   Getting to know you: This includes obtaining personal information about life before the individual became ill, their likes and dislikes, obstacles to communicating, what they are feeling currently and what the communicating partner feels when they try to interact.
2   Consideration of the communication environment: for example how often does someone interact with the person on a daily basis, what type of communication most often occurs
3   Recognising the fundamentals of communication as reflected in eye gaze, facial expression, speech / speech sounds, sounds, physical contact, gestures, imitation, bodily position, emotion and turn taking. While not specifically mentioned by Ellis and Astell, tuning into the elderly adult's rhythms (e.g., of their articulations or breathing patterns) also offers opportunities for the beginnings of engagement and shared communication (Ellis and Astell, 2018, pp. 172–176).

Intensive Interaction and responsive communication

Sensory abnormalities have long been recognised in autism (Leekam et al., 2007) and are now considered a diagnostic feature (DSM-5) (American Psychiatric Association, 2013). Neural underpinnings are described (Marco et al., 2011). Many behaviours that challenge (anything from self injury, aggression directed towards others, meltdowns, avoidance and social withdrawal) seen in autism are associated with these hyper- and hypo-sensory sensitivities and processing differences. Using body language (Intensive Interaction) to get in touch with children and adults with autism engaging in such behaviours highlights the impact of different sensory experiences and processing in causing stress and triggering anxiety (Caldwell, 2014, Caldwell et al., 2019; Caldwell and Zutt, 2022). For example, a sensory environment where the individual's specific sensory hypersensitivity is triggered can seriously delay (or even prohibit) the effectiveness of attempted interactions. These triggers may not be immediately apparent or recognised; for example, the care provider's black and white striped top (visual trigger) or their particular body or mouth odour (olfactory trigger) causing distress to the individual with visual or olfactory hyper-sensitivity. Only the concerning behaviour is observed and not the trigger. Such sensitivities can be present in any of our sensory domains e.g., olfactory, visual, auditory, gustatory, vestibular and tactile, as well as emotional.

In optimising Intensive Interaction encounters, Caldwell identifies the need to: (a) observe an individual's experience of sensory inputs; (b) identify which inputs cause distress or discomfort, which are neutral or positive; and from this (c) create an autism-friendly environment by: reducing or eliminating sensory inputs that are causing the person distress (i.e., inputs to which they are hyper-sensitive) and increasing those sensory inputs which they experience as positive or to which they are hypo- or under-sensitive. Additionally, responding to emotional affect (how the person is feeling) and validating their emotional experience engages shared attention. *Responsive communication* refers to Intensive Interaction embedded in this appreciation, by the communicating partner, of both the emotional and sensory world from the perspective of the individual with autism (Caldwell, 2018a, 2018b; The Caldwell Autism Foundation, 2017).

Music and emotional engagement

Music, like body language, can also facilitate the sharing of emotions, intentions and meanings, even though spoken language may be mutually incomprehensible (MacDonald, 2008). Singing and early reciting of nursery rhythms by the primary care provider have been linked to emotional and mental integration through rhythmic attunement between infant and care provider, contributing to the regulation of vital states of the body (e.g., cardiac vagal tone) (Trevarthen, 2009). As noted previously, tuning in and responding to rhythms and patterns of articulations and body movements (e.g., breathing pattern) are often ways to make connection with a seemingly otherwise self-absorbed individual. Rhythms and patterns are also "recognised" across sensory systems; sometimes the "surprise" (or "jolt") consequent to the communicating partner responding to an individual's rhythm or pattern of expression using a different sensory system, is needed to capture and fix the individual's attention on something outside of this self-absorption. For example, responding to the individual's articulation rhythm by scratching on a surface rather than by a responsive vocalisation.

How applicable are these observations and non-verbal approaches working with individuals with IDD and ASD (some of whom may also meet criteria for psychosis), to those with psychosis without IDD or autism? This begs the question "what is psychosis?" and touches upon the extent to which psychosis, ASD and IDD share similarities or overlap.

What is psychosis?

Psychosis (or psychotic) is a general umbrella term for a wide variety of conditions where the individual is described as losing touch with reality as manifested by delusions, hallucinations, or disorganised thinking, accompanied by disorganised or catatonic behaviour or negative symptoms. Psychotic symptoms, the cardinal feature in schizophrenia and other psychotic disorders (DSM-5) are also described in other mental health disorders (e.g., mood disorder, Trauma- and Stressor-Related Disorders), associated with some medical conditions (e.g., Alzheimer's, Parkinson's, hypoglycaemia, multiple sclerosis) and with substance misuse (e.g., cocaine, LSD, as a side effect, or overdose, of some prescribed medications) (NHS – Choices UK, 2016). Psychosis, in vulnerable individuals, is associated with social stress (e.g., marginalisation, victimisation, discrimination, social defeat, childhood abuse and trauma, cumulative life events) (Mizrahi, 2016; van Winkel, Stefanis and Myin-Germeys, 2008). A positive relationship between loneliness and psychosis has been confirmed by a meta-analysis review (Michalska da Rocha et al., 2018); psychotic experiences are described in sleep disruption (Reeve et al., 2017) and sensory deprivation (Daniel, Lovatt and Mason, 2014) also. Hearing voices (auditory verbal hallucinations) are now recognised as being relatively common in non-clinical populations (Upthegrove et al., 2016) from childhood through to old age (de Leede-Smith and Barkus, 2013; Longden, Madill and Waterman, 2012); such experiences may worsen with anxiety and loneliness (Lim and Gleeson, 2014).

Psychotic disorders, IDD and ASD

Schizophrenia is the most severe and enduring form of psychotic disorder. Ongoing research of aetiological (i.e., genetic and developmental) circumstances, suggests that schizophrenia and other psychotic disorders might be better understood as a spectrum of related disorders (SSD) along a neurodevelopmental continuum (that includes other developmental disorders such as IDD, ASD, ADHD) rather than as a separate entity (Owen and O'Donovan, 2017); or as the end point of a cascade of neurodevelopmental risk factors interfacing with adverse social and drug risk factors (Murray et al., 2017).

Adverse life events, abuse and trauma are increasingly being recognised in the lives of people with IDD (Wigham, Taylor and Hatton, 2014). Early traumas in the lives of some adults diagnosed with SSD have also been identified, a finding that has given rise to a Traumagenic Neurodevelopmental model of SSD (Read et al., 2014). Greater understanding of genetic and environmental causes of SSD is offering opportunities to alter its course: for example, interventions for social isolation and vulnerability to psychological stress as these have been identified as significant risks in prodromal symptoms transitioning to SSD (Millan et al., 2016). Psychotic episodes in of themselves are also described as being traumatising (Rodrigues and Anderson, 2017). An ongoing circumstance in the lives of many with ASD also described as being extremely distressing and to be avoided, if at all possible, is that of "meltdowns" associated with being overwhelmed by some daily challenges and expectations beyond their capabilities (Lipsky, 2011).

The psychological consequences of trauma not infrequently contribute to diagnostic uncertainty between these neurodevelopmental disorders (namely ASD, IDD and SSD), as trauma-related symptomatology and behaviours (Trauma-Related Stress Disorders [TRSD] – DSM-5) (American Psychiatric Association, 2013) overlap with diagnostic features of SSD (McCarthy-Jones and Longden, 2015). For example, hearing voices may occur in dissociation, the latter a characteristic of TRSD; but auditory hallucinations are also characteristic of SSD (Hamner, 2011; Lindley, Carlson and Sheikh, 2000); likewise catatonic behaviours previously considered a characteristic only of SSD have also been described in individuals with ASD (Wing and Shah, 2000; Wing and Shah, 2006).

Sensory differences in ASD are recognised in diagnostic criteria for ASD (DSM-5) and are found to be underpinned by neurophysiological correlates (Marco et al., 2011). Along the continuum of psychosis, differences in sensory processing (Javitt, 2009; Javitt and Freedman, 2015), integration (Carter et al., 2017), underpinned by neurophysiological correlates (Javitt and Freedman, 2015; Carter et al., 2017; Andrade et al., 2016), are also being identified (Carter et al., 2017; Randeniya, Oestreich and Garrido, 2018). People experiencing psychosis report being hypersensitive to sensory experiences (Javitt and Freedman, 2015; Smucny et al., 2013; Light and Braff, 2000); these hypersensitivities and sensory processing differences (e.g., sensory prediction errors) (Randeniya, Oestreich and Garrido, 2018) are being linked to the experience of positive symptoms (e.g., hallucinations, perceptual distortions) (Carter et al., 2017). Such differences in sensory reception and processing have implications for intervention (Marco et al., 2011; Javitt, 2009; Javitt and Freedman, 2015).

Sensory issues in SSD are still not widely recognised in clinical practice. However, the impact of emotional connection and personal relationships has been recognised in understanding relapse prevention in SSD (Expressed Emotion) (Leff, 1985; Leff and Vaughn, 1985) and these are embodied in one approach to manage symptoms (Avatar therapy) (Craig et al., 2018; Box 1).

Emotional connection in (a) the treatment of schizophrenia and (b) auditory hallucinations

a. Expressed Emotion

Expressed emotion (EE) refers to several categories of emotional response identified in family members of the individual with SSD: critical comments, hostility, warmth and overinvolvement. Considerable attention is paid to the vocal aspects of speech use by relatives (e.g., rate, volume, and pitch) as ratings of relatives' EE have been found to depend not only on what is said, but also on the way in which it is expressed (Leff, 1985). High ratings of EE are associated with greater tendency to relapse (Leff and Vaughn, 1985). Working with families and other care providers to reduce such negative emotional milieux and responses is associated with better outcomes.

b. Avatar therapy (Leff et al., 2014)

Avatar therapy is a method to facilitate a dialogue between the voice hearer and the entity they believe to be speaking to them, by enabling the patient to create an avatar of the entity, human or non-human.

The patient constructs the avatar, using the computer software to choose a face and a voice that approximates to the entity they hear. The range of voices from which the patient chooses is produced by morphing the therapist's voice into a variety of forms. This enables the therapist to speak to the patient through the avatar in real time using the selected voice.

The patient sits in a room and faces a monitor on which their avatar is shown. The avatar's lip movements are synchronised with its speech by the software. The therapist sits in an adjacent room and views a screen. Clicking on the right side of the screen allows the therapist to speak to the patient through the avatar using the morphed voice. Clicking on the left side of the screen enables the therapist to speak to the patient in their normal voice.

The patient is prompted to enter into a dialogue with their avatar and encouraged to oppose it. The therapist controls the avatar so that it gradually comes under the patient's control over six weekly sessions of 30 minutes duration.

Over the course of the therapy the avatar progressively changes from being persecutory to becoming appreciative and supportive. Each session is digitally recorded and the audio file transferred to a personal media player which is given to the patients to use at any time to reinforce their control over the persecutory "voice".

Excerpt from Leff et al. (2014) with permission from Julian Leff, 3 April 2018

Trauma therapists and researchers have shown how our sense of ourselves is anchored in a vital connection with our bodies (van der Kolk, 2014). While trauma may be a thing of the past, the body keeps reacting as if it is still in imminent danger. From this perspective, treatment of psychosis associated with trauma will likely involve learning how to tolerate painful memories and not be overwhelmed by them. A vital part of knowing our bodies comes through interoception. While proprioception is awareness of our body in relation to external objects, and exteroception awareness of stimuli coming from outside our bodies (e.g., visual, auditory, tactile, olfactory), interoception is awareness of what goes on within the boundaries of our skin (Emerson, 2015). Afferent (sensory) homeostatic fibres conduct information about the physiological state of the body including mechanical, thermal, chemical, metabolic and hormonal information from the skin, muscles, joints and visceral tissues, to the interoceptive cortex in the brain called the insula (limbic sensory cortex). The insula thus carries a distinct cortical image of the physiological condition of the body: "the material me" (Craig, 2002). This interoceptive neural system is associated with autonomic motor control through the anterior cingulate gyrus (limbic motor cortex), working to maintain the body in homeostasis. Functional imaging brain studies demonstrate subjective feelings (e.g., emotions, moods) correlated with interoceptive cortical activity (Craig, 2003), i.e., subjective awareness and "the feeling me".

Summary

Treating psychosis (whether this is associated with SSD, ASD, ID or trauma) with respect, involves emotional engagement between two people (a relational therapy): the individual with psychosis and a resonating empathetic other (the therapist) to support the individual through the journey of integrating fragmented parts of the self: the "material me" and the "feeling me", past and present. Attunement through the language of the individual, whether this is nonverbal (e.g., Intensive Interaction) or verbal (e.g., Avatar therapy), confirms for the individual the integrity of their emotional and psychological experiences, empowers them to maintain connection with their feeling body (interoception) and supports them in beginning to experience, without fear, their bodily reactions (self-regulation). The therapist provides a therapeutic space attentive to sensory (e.g., hyper- and hypo-sensory sensitivities) emotional (e.g., not intruding, not imposing) and safety (trust, expectations that do not overwhelm) needs. The addition of simple "invitational" language describing and demonstrating physical movements that the individual may follow (such as in trauma-sensitive yoga practices [Emerson, 2015] – an evidence-based trauma treatment), may encourage and empower individuals (even those with few words), to join in, thus offering them the opportunity to experience their own (functional) body in a safe environment with an empathic other.

Conclusion

> If there is one lesson that I have learned during my life as an analyst, it is the lesson that what my patients tell me is likely to be true — that many times when I believed that I was right and my patients were wrong, it turned out, though often only after a prolonged search, that **my** rightness was superficial and **their** rightness was profound.
>
> (Kohut, Goldberg and Stepansky, 1984, p. 93, emphasis in original)

With the above written in 1984, we may think we have by now learned to listen to our patients. But how do we know? How for example do we listen and tune into sensory experiences and perceptions experienced by others that may be foreign or unknown to us? Kish, a blind man who navigates the world through echolocation, eloquently shares his perspective:

> blindness is a state of mind ... our [those with blindness] goal is to help everyone see more clearly to greater freedom ... blind individuals learning to see (for example by echolocation) can serve an illustrative example to everyone ... that we are all challenged by blindness in our lives ... psychological blindness, social blindness, spiritual blindness ... the most debilitating, dangerous form of blindness is blindness to our own blindness.
>
> (Kish, 2015)

Caldwell offers some guidance in how we might overcome our own blindness to experiences of others that are not immediately our own:

> In order to build in empathy to my responses, I need to use all my senses to tune into the affective quality of their activity. I need to feel what they feel in my own bones. First of all, I empty myself and place myself entirely at my partner's disposal.
>
> (Caldwell, 2008, p. 171)

Bibliography

American Psychiatric Association. (2013). *Diagnostic and Statistical Manual of Mental Disorders: DSM-5*. 5th Edn. Arlington, VI: American Psychiatric Association.

Andrade, G.N., Butler, J.S., Peters, G.A., Molholm, S. and Foxe, J.J. (2016). Atypical visual and somatosensory adaptation in schizophrenia-spectrum disorders. *Translational Psychiatry*, **6**e804. Available at: https://www.ncbi.nlm.nih.gov/pmc/articles/PMC5070065/ (accessed 2018).

Andrew, E.M., Gray, N.S. and Snowden, R.J. (2008). The relationship between trauma and beliefs about hearing voices: A study of psychiatric and non-psychiatric voice hearers. *Psychological Medicine*, 38 (10), 1409–1417.

Beebe, B. and Lachmann, F.M. (1988). Mother-infant mutual influence and precursors of psychic structure. In A. Goldberg (ed.), *Progress in Self Psychology, vol 3: Frontiers in Self Psychology*, 3–25. Hillsdale, NJ: Analytic Press.

Beebe, B. (2014). My journey in infant research and psychoanalysis: Microanalysis, a social microscope. *Psychoanalytic Psychology*, 31(1), 4–25. Available at: https://www.apa.org/pubs/journals/features/pap-a0035575.pdf (accessed 2018).

Beebe, B., Lachmann, F. and Jaffe, J. (1997). Mother-infant interaction structures and presymbolic self- and object representations. *Psychoanalytic Dialogues*, 7(2), 133–182.

Bradley, E., Caldwell, P. and Underwood, L. (2014). Autism spectrum disorder. In E. Tsakanikos and J. McCarthy (Eds) *Handbook of Psychopathology in Intellectual Disability: Research, Practice and Policy,* 237–264. New York, Heidelberg:Springer.

Brendel, R.W. and Stern, T.A. (2005). Psychotic symptoms in the elderly. *Primary Care Companion to the Journal of Clinical Psychiatry*, 7(5), 238–241. Available at: https://www.ncbi.nlm.nih.gov/pmc/articles/PMC1257410/ (accessed 2018).

Bruner, J. (2014). *How does teaching influence learning?* Available from: https://www.youtube.com/watch?v=aljvAuXqhds (accessed 2018).

Buber, M. and Kaufmann, W.A. (1970). *I and Thou*. New York: Scribner,

Caldwell, P. (2007). *Learning the Language – Gabriel*. Brighton, England: Pavilion Publishing and Media Ltd.

Caldwell, P. (2018a). Responsive Communication and autism. Available at Intellectual Disability and Health, University of Hertfordshire, UK. https://www.intellectualdisability.info/how-to-guides/articles/responsive-communication-and-autism accessed on 25 May 2025

Caldwell, P. (2018b). Responsive Communication: Tuning in to people with autism. Video # 2 Gabriel, available from https://phoebecaldwell.com/videos (accessed 11 February 2024).

Caldwell, P. (2018c). Responsive Communication: Tuning in to people with autism. Video # 24 Pranve, available from https://phoebecaldwell.com/videos (accessed 11 February 2024).

Caldwell, P. (2014). *The Anger Box: Sensory Turmoil and Pain in Autism*. Hove, East Sussex, United Kingdom: Pavilion Publishing and Media Ltd.

Caldwell, P., Bradley, E., Gurney, J., Heath, J., Lightowler, H., Richardson, K. and Swales, J. (2019). *Responsive Communication: Combining Attention to Sensory Issues with Using Body Language (Intensive Interaction) to Interact with Autistic Adults and Children*. Hove, East Sussex, United Kingdom: Pavilion Publishing and Media Ltd.

Caldwell, P. and Zutt, Z. (2022). *Autism: Respecting Difference. An Inside View of Autism for Carers, Professionals and Families*. Hove, East Sussex, United Kingdom: Pavilion Publishing and Media Ltd.

Caldwell, P. (2012). *Intensive Interaction – Films – An Intervention with Jamie* [*excerpt 3:53 min at site*]. Available from: https ://phoebecaldwell.com/visual-training-ganhu (accessed 11 February 2024).

Caldwell, P. (2008). Intensive Interaction: Getting in touch with a child with severe autism. In M.S. Zeedyk (Ed.), *Promoting Social Interaction for Individuals with Communicative Impairments: Making Contact*, 170–184. London, England: Jessica Kingsley Publishers.

Carter, O., Bennett, D., Nash, T., Arnold, S., Brown, L., Cai R.Y., Allan, Z., Dluzniak, A., McAnally K., Burr, D. and Sundram S. (2017). Sensory integration deficits support a dimensional view of psychosis and are not limited to schizophrenia. *Translational Psychiatry*, 7(5), e1118. Available at: https://www.ncbi.nlm.nih.gov/pmc/articles/PMC5534945/ (accessed 2018).

Craig, A.D. (2003). Interoception: The sense of the physiological condition of the body. *Current Opinion in Neurobiology*, 13(4), 500–505.

Craig, A.D. (2002). How do you feel? Interoception: The sense of the physiological condition of the body. *Nature Reviews. Neuroscience*, 3(8), 655–666.

Craig, T.K., Rus-Calafell, M., Ward, T., Leff, J.P., Huckvale, M., Howarth, E., Emsley, R. and Garety, P.A. (2018). AVATAR therapy for auditory verbal hallucinations in people with psychosis: A single-blind, randomised controlled trial. *Lancet Psychiatry*, 5(1), 31–40.

Daniel, C., Lovatt, A. and Mason, O.J. (2014). Psychotic-like experiences and their cognitive appraisal under short-term sensory deprivation. *Frontiers in Psychiatry*, 5, 106. Available at: https://www.ncbi.nlm.nih.gov/pmc/articles/PMC4133754/ (accessed 2018).

Davies, C.E., Zeedyk, M.S., Walls, S., Betts, N. and Parry, S. (2008). Using imitation to establish channels of communication with institutionalised children in Romania: Bridging the gap. In M.S. Zeedyk (ed.), *Promoting Social Interaction for Individuals with Communicative Impairments: Making Contact,* 84–101. London, England: Jessica Kingsley Publishers.

Davis, D.R. (2015). Moments of meeting: A self psychological approach. *International Journal of Psychoanalytic Self Psychology*, 10(1), 69–79.

de Leede-Smith, S. and Barkus, E. (2013). A comprehensive review of auditory verbal hallucinations: Lifetime prevalence, correlates and mechanisms in healthy and clinical individuals. *Frontiers in Human Neuroscience*, 7 Article 367. Available at: https://www.ncbi.nlm.nih.gov/pmc/articles/PMC3712258/ (accessed 2018).

Ellis, M., and Astell, A. (2018). *Adaptive Interaction and Dementia: How to Communicate Without Speech.* Illustrations by S. Scott. London; Philadelphia: Jessica Kingsley Publishers.

Emerson, D. (2015). *Trauma-Sensitive Yoga in Therapy: Bringing the Body into Treatment.* New York: W.W. Norton and Company.

Ephraim, G. (1990). *A Brief Introduction to Augmented Mothering: Giving a Person with Severe and Complex Learning Difficulties Control Over Her World.* Harperbury Hospital, Radlett: Playtrac.

Federici, R.S. (1998). *Help for the Hopeless Child: A Guide for Families: With Special Discussion for Assessing and Treating the Post-Institutionalized Child.* Alexandria, VI: Ronald S. Federici and Associates.

Garrett, M. and Silva, R. (2003). Auditory hallucinations, source monitoring, and the belief that "voices" are real. *Schizophrenia Bulletin*, 29(3), 445–457.

Grandin, T. and Duffy, K. (2008). *Developing Talents: Careers for Individuals with Asperger Syndrome and High-Functioning Autism.* Shawnee Mission, KS: Autism Asperger Pub. Co.

Hamner, M.B. (2011). Psychotic symptoms in posttraumatic stress disorder. *FOC*, 9 (3), 278–285.

Hart, P. (2008). Sharing communicative landscapes with congenitally deafblind people: It's a walk in the park! In M.S. Zeedyk (ed.), *Promoting Social Interaction for Individuals with Communicative Impairments: Making Contact.* London, England: Jessica Kingsley Publishers, 66–83.

Javitt, D.C. (2009). Sensory processing in schizophrenia: neither simple nor intact. *Schizophrenia Bulletin*, 35(6), 1059–1064.

Javitt, D.C. and Freedman R. (2015). Sensory processing dysfunction in the personal experience and neuronal machinery of schizophrenia. *The American Journal of Psychiatry*, 172(1), 17–31.

Kish, D. (2012). Teaching the blind to navigate the world using tongue clicks: Daniel Kish at TEDxGateway 2012 [Video]. Available at: https://www.youtube.com/watch?v=ob-P2a6Mrjs (accessed July 9 2025).

Kitwood, T. (1997). The experience of dementia. *Aging and Mental Health*, 1(1), 13–22.

Knudsen, E.I. (2002). Instructed learning in the auditory localization pathway of the barn owl. *Nature*, 417(6886), 322–328.

Kohut, H., Goldberg, A. and Stepansky, P.E. (1984). *How Does Analysis Cure?* Chicago, IL: University of Chicago Press.

Kolvin, I. (1971). Studies in the childhood psychoses. I. Diagnostic criteria and classification. *The British Journal of Psychiatry*, 118(545), 381–384.

Leekam, S.R., Nieto, C., Libby, S.J., Wing L. and Gould, J. (2007). Describing the sensory abnormalities of children and adults with autism. *Journal of Autism and Developmental Disorders*, 37(5), 894–910.

Leff, J. (1985). The concepts of expressed emotion: New empirical evidence. In P. Pichot, P. Berner, R. Wolf and K. Thau (eds), *Epidemiology and Community Psychiatry*, 501–507. Boston, MS: Springer.

Leff, J., Williams, G., Huckvale M., Arbuthnot, M. and Leff A.P. (2014). Avatar therapy for persecutory auditory hallucinations: What is it and how does it work? *Psychosis*, 6(2), 166–176.

Leff, J.P. and Vaughn, C. (1985). *Expressed Emotion in Families: Its Significance for Mental Illness*. New York: Guilford Press.

Light, G.A. and Braff, D.L. (2000). Do self-reports of perceptual anomalies reflect gating deficits in schizophrenia patients? *Biological Psychiatry*, 47(5), 463–467.

Lim, M.H. and Gleeson, J.F. (2014). Social connectedness across the psychosis spectrum: current issues and future directions for interventions in loneliness. *Frontiers in Psychiatry*, 5, 154.

Lindley, S.E., Carlson, E. and Sheikh, J. (2000). Psychotic symptoms in posttraumatic stress disorder. *CNS Spectrums*, 5(9), 52–57.

Lipsky, D. (2011). *From Anxiety to Meltdown: How Individuals on the Autism Spectrum Deal with Anxiety, Experience Meltdowns, Manifest Tantrums, and How You Can Intervene Effectively*. London; Philadelphia: Jessica Kingsley Publishers.

Longden, E., Madill, A. and Waterman, M.G. (2012). Dissociation, trauma, and the role of lived experience: Toward a new conceptualization of voice hearing. *Psychological Bulletin*, 138(1), 28–76.

MacDonald, R.A.R. (2008). The universality of musical communication. In M.S. Zeedyk (ed.), *Promoting Social Interaction for Individuals with Communicative Impairments: Making Contact*, 39–50. London, England: Jessica Kingsley Publishers.

Marco, E.J., Hinkley, L.B., Hill, S.S. and Nagarajan, S.S. (2011). Sensory processing in autism: A review of neurophysiologic findings. *Pediatric Research*, 69(5 Pt. 2), 48R-54R.

McCarthy-Jones, S. and Longden, E. (2015). Auditory verbal hallucinations in schizophrenia and post-traumatic stress disorder: Common phenomenology, common cause, common interventions? *Frontiers in Psychology*, 6(July 28), 1071. Available at: https://www.ncbi.nlm.nih.gov/pmc/articles/PMC4517448/ (accessed May 19 2018).

Michalska da Rocha, B., Rhodes, S., Vasilopoulou, E. and Hutton, P. (2018). Loneliness in psychosis: A meta-analytical review. *Schizophrenia Bulletin*, 44(1), 114–125.

Millan, M.J., Andrieux, A., Bartzokis, G., Cadenhead, K., Dazzan, P., Fusar-Poli, P., Gallinat, J., Giedd, J., Grayson, D.R., Heinrichs, M., Kahn, R., Krebs, M.O., Leboyer, M., Lewis, D., Marin, O., Marin, P., Meyer-Lindenberg, A., McGorry, P., McGuire, P., Owen, M.J., Patterson, P., Sawa, A., Spedding, M., Uhlhaas, P., Vaccarino, F., Wahlestedt, C. and Weinberger, D. (2016). Altering the course of schizophrenia: Progress and perspectives. *Nature Reviews Drug Discovery*, 15(7), 485–515.

Mizrahi, R. (2016). Social stress and psychosis risk: Common neurochemical substrates? *Neuropsychopharmacology*, 41(3), 666–674. Available at: https://www.ncbi.nlm.nih.gov/pmc/articles/PMC4707841/ (accessed 2018).

Murray, R.M., Bhavsar, V., Tripoli, G. and Howes, O. (2017). 30 Years on: How the neurodevelopmental hypothesis of schizophrenia morphed into the developmental risk factor model of psychosis. *Schizophrenia Bulletin*, 43(6), 1190–1196.

NHS – Choices UK (2016). *Psychosis – causes*. Available from: https://www.nhs.uk/conditions/psychosis/causes/ (accessed 2018).

Nind, M. and Hewett, D. (1994). *Access to Communication: Developing the Basics of Communication with People with Severe Learning Difficulties Through Intensive Interaction*. London: D. Fulton.

Owen, M.J. and O'Donovan, M.C. (2017). Schizophrenia and the neurodevelopmental continuum: Evidence from genomics. *World Psychiatry: Official Journal of the World Psychiatric Association (WPA)*, 16(3), 227–235. Available at: https://www.ncbi.nlm.nih.gov/pmc/articles/PMC5608820/ (accessed 2018).

Randeniya, R., Oestreich, L.K.L. and Garrido, M.I. (2018). Sensory prediction errors in the continuum of psychosis. *Schizophrenia Research*, 191, 109–122.

Read, J., Fosse, R., Moskowitz, A. and Perry, B. (2014). The traumagenic neurodevelopmental model of psychosis revisited. *Neuropsychiatry*, 4(1), 65–79. Available at: http://www.jneuropsychiatry.org/peer-review/the-traumagenic-neurodevelopmental-model-of-psychosis-revisited-neuropsychiatry.pdf (accessed 2018).

Reeve, S., Emsley, R., Sheaves, B. and Freeman, D. (2017). Disrupting sleep: The effects of sleep loss on psychotic experiences tested in an experimental study with mediation analysis. *Schizophrenia Bulletin*, 44(3), 662–671. Available at: https://www.ncbi.nlm.nih.gov/pmc/articles/PMC5890488/ (accessed 2018).

Rodrigues, R. and Anderson, K.K. (2017). The traumatic experience of first-episode psychosis: A systematic review and meta-analysis. *Schizophrenia Research*, 189, 27–36.

Rutter, M. (1972). Childhood schizophrenia reconsidered. *Journal of Autism and Childhood Schizophrenia*, 2(4), 315–337.

Rutter, M., Andersen-Wood, L., Beckett, C., Bredenkamp, D., Castle, J., Groothues, C., Kreppner, J., Keaveney, L., Lord, C. and O'Connor, T.G. (1999). Quasi-autistic patterns following severe early global privation. English and Romanian Adoptees (ERA) Study Team. *Journal of Child Psychology and Psychiatry, and Allied Disciplines*, 40(4), 537–549.

Rutter, M.L., Kreppner, J.M., O'Connor, T.G. and English and Romanian Adoptees (ERA) study team (2001). Specificity and heterogeneity in children's responses to profound institutional privation. *The British Journal of Psychiatry*, 17997–103.

Smucny, J., Rojas, D.C., Eichman, L.C. and Tregellas, J.R. (2013). Neural effects of auditory distraction on visual attention in schizophrenia. *PloS One*, 8(4), e60606.

Spitz, R.A. (1945). Hospitalism; an inquiry into the genesis of psychiatric conditions in early childhood. *The Psychoanalytic Study of the Child*, 1, 53–74.

Stern, D.N. (1985). *The Interpersonal World of the Infant: A View from Psychoanalysis and Developmental Psychology*. New York: Basic Books.

The CaldwellAutism Foundation (2017). *Responsive Communication Pilot Project*. More information available at https://www.autismwellbeing.org.uk/ (accessed May 2025).

Trevarthen, C. and Delafield-Butt, J.T. (2017). Intersubjectivity in the imagination and feelings of the infant: Implications for education in the early years. In E.J. White and C. Dalli (eds), *Under-Three Year Olds in Policy and Practice,* 17–39. New York, NY: Springer.

Trevarthen, C. (2016). *Pre-birth to three: Professor Colwyn Trevarthen - Relationships* [*4:38 min*]. Available from: https://www.youtube.com/watch?v=2kJI6G35TNk (accessed 2018).

Trevarthen, C. (2014). *Remembering Daniel Stern.* Available from: https://blog.oup.com/2014/01/remembering-daniel-stern-developmental-psychologist/ (accessed 2018).

Trevarthen, C. (2013). *Visions of infant joy.* Birthright Conference2006 [9:09 min]. Available from: https://www.youtube.com/watch?v=iwc4iwRmA3U (accessed April 21 2018).

Trevarthen C. (2009). Human biochronology: On the source and functions of 'musicality'. In R. Haas and V. Brandes (eds), *Music That Works: Contributions of Biology, Neurophysiology, Psychology, Sociology, Medicine and Musicology,* 221–265. Vienna: Springer.

Trevarthen C. (2008). Intuition for human communication. In M.S. Zeedyk (ed.), *Promoting Social Interaction for Individuals with Communicative Impairments: Making Contact,* 221–265. London, England: Jessica Kingsley Publishers.

Upthegrove, R., Broome, M.R., Caldwell, K., Ives, J., Oyebode, F. and Wood S.J. (2016). Understanding auditory verbal hallucinations: A systematic review of current evidence. *Acta Psychiatrica Scandinavica,* 133(5), 352–367.

Van der Kolk, B.A. (2014). *The Body Keeps the Score: Brain, Mind, and Body in the Healing of Trauma.* New York: Viking.

van Winkel, R., Stefanis, N.C. and Myin-Germeys, I. (2008). Psychosocial stress and psychosis. A review of the neurobiological mechanisms and the evidence for gene-stress interaction. *Schizophrenia Bulletin,* 34(6), 1095–1105.

Wigham, S., Taylor, J.L. and Hatton, C. (2014). A prospective study of the relationship between adverse life events and trauma in adults with mild to moderate intellectual disabilities. *Journal of Intellectual Disability Research,* 58(12), 1131–1140.

Wing, L. and Shah, A. (2006). A systematic examination of catatonia-like clinical pictures in autism spectrum disorders. *International Review of Neurobiology,* 72, 21–39.

Wing, L. and Shah, A. (2000). Catatonia in autistic spectrum disorders. *The British Journal of Psychiatry,* 176, 357–362.

Woods, A. (2017). On shame and voice-hearing. *Medical Humanities,* 43(4), 251–256.

Woods, A., Jones N., Alderson-Day B., Callard, F. and Fernyhough C. (2015). Experiences of hearing voices: Analysis of a novel phenomenological survey. *Lancet Psychiatry,* 2(4), 323–331. Available at: https://www.ncbi.nlm.nih.gov/pmc/articles/PMC4580735/ (accessed 2018).

Zeedyk, M.S. (n.d.) "*Connected Baby*" – https://connectedbaby.net (accessed 2018).

Zeedyk, M.S. (2008). *Promoting Social Interaction for Individuals with Communicative Impairments: Making Contact.* London, England: Jessica Kingsley Publishers.

Chapter 13

Therapy with Dr Alan Corbett

François Marshall and Marvin Marshall-Springer

This chapter goes to the core of the clinical experience. It provides a first-person lived experience account of the psychotherapeutic support offered by Dr Alan Corbett to Marvin and François as carers of James. It details successful individual therapy that moved into couples and then family psychotherapy with Alan Corbett. 'James' was a courageous but profoundly traumatised young man who was aided by a remarkable older couple, Marvin and François. Together, they faced the lack of understanding of local services and the enormous toll it took on them to fight for, and finally find, the right therapy for James and themselves. 'James' was othered with Dissociative Identity Disorder in the same way patients with an intellectual disability are and Alan Corbett, like many of our key disability therapists recognised this and worked with it. This chapter provides an emotionally direct account of how Dr Alan Corbett worked and the impact he had.

Introduction

In January 2010, we started caring for a friend, James, that was going through what looked to us like a 'mental health emergency'. Marvin had initially met him five years earlier when working in the north of England for a few months, and we had become friends. James was 19 and had ambitions to become a fine painting artist. We effectively ended up taking him under our wings. Over time we started suspecting that all was not well with his mental health – but the breakdown at the start of 2010 was of a different magnitude. We stepped in, in what we thought to be a temporary intervention, until 'the authorities' took over and adequate help was dispensed (a naive assumption in retrospect). What actually followed was a multi-year project, that fully took over our lives. But at no point could we contemplate walking away as we feared that without our care and support his recovery would never materialise, and worse, would probably come to an abrupt, premature end.

The first year was gruelling. Marvin moved to the north of England to care for James full time and was determined to get him the appropriate compassionate help he needed. François carried on working in London during the week and would travel up on the weekend. Initially James was offered to

DOI: 10.4324/9781003646242-17

attend a local 'acute community service' during the day (now closed). This was better than nothing, but this centre was not dispensing any forms of talking therapy. It was running cooking classes and board games etc., simply trying to keep its patients distracted. Most of the patients were known to the service and would come in and out as if through a revolving door. However, one of the mental health nurses working there took an interest in his case and suggested he could be suffering from dissociative identity disorder (DID). There he was also prescribed anti-psychotic drugs, as a starting point.

A carers' support charity offered Marvin some weekly counselling, which was a lifeline given how stressful the situation was. At the same time Marvin desperately navigated the maze of mental health services trying to get a firm diagnosis for James. The acute community service, after running several tests and assessments, was very reluctant to narrow down the diagnosis. Several hypotheses were put forward – psycho-affective disorder, schizophrenia, DID. The case was then passed on to another local mental health charity, who also were not committing to a single diagnosis. Marvin, based on his interaction with James, and the training he had sought independently about dissociation, was convinced that James was suffering from DID and had selected the Clinic of Dissociative Studies (CDS), in London, as the way forward. We also asked James's psychiatrist to stop the anti-psychotic drugs, given they are not clinically recommended for DID sufferers.

The road to getting a fully approved treatment package for James however was very tortuous, and frankly traumatising. Many tense meetings with different bodies and people were required. Most professionals Marvin saw lacked empathy and appeared indifferent to James's experience. And initially the request was denied – it looked as if James would not be treated. Through a Carers Week Marvin had met the head of the local NHS trust, so he appealed to him directly. A kind and extremely helpful man, his intervention helped to get the case reviewed and eventually a treatment package for DID at the CDS was approved.

An extremely difficult period started however. As the effect from the anti-psychotic drugs lifted, James started remembering the details of the historical sexual abuse he suffered as a child, and how he was sexually exploited by his biological mother. The start of treatment at the CDS, set for January 2011, could not come fast enough, as our family unit was now filled with daily accounts of depraved and sickening abuse. It had taken almost a year to get to that point, a year supporting James as best we could, but without the specialised therapeutic help that was required. The package, to our surprise, would include weekly support therapy for Marvin, as the primary carer.

Marvin's first experiences with Alan

First fifteen

I remember the day I first met Alan. It must have been February or March 2011. To be honest I did not like him initially! On the way to the session, I had just been pulled over by police for driving whilst on the phone. That call I took was from James, threatening to commit suicide. I had argued with the police officer (unsuccessfully), that the only reason I took the call was to save somebody's life. I arrived dishevelled and extremely late for my session, having only 15 mins left of my allotted time. To my horror and to my naive surprise, Alan ended the session on time. This did not go down well in my estimations. Truly he could not care about what I was going through. I put him in that long list of health and care professionals that really had little empathy.

Having decided I didn't like him, I was still determined to get from him any knowledge that I could. Looking back now, I can clearly see that Alan by ending the session at the normal time was setting boundaries and ensuring that his own schedule was not disrupted. Nevertheless, I kept attending the weekly sessions. There was a lot to cover, as James's condition was still far from stable (as the incident on the very first session proved), and his outbursts were frequent and very devastating. James would routinely self-harm, medicate with alcohol. He could be violent too, attacking me physically on a few occasions.

I had a lot of rage and resentment about how my life had been taken over, and how I felt I had to care for him, 24/7. As I write this, I am triggered still by the sheer chaos and how powerless I felt, something that echoed my own dysfunctional childhood home – something I had sworn to myself I would never replicate in my adult life.

We also spent a lot of time in the early months to further my understanding of DID, and how to best manage James day to day. This training was on top of earlier conversations with other clinic staff at the CDS.

Fight

The year leading to the referral to the CDS had put me in contact with many people from social services, mental health teams, the NHS etc. There were a handful of outstanding people, but many felt indifferent to James's case, some were clearly incompetent and out of their depth, and a very few were mean-spirited, a disturbing thought when considering they would be interacting with the most vulnerable in society. In all interactions it felt like I had to bludgeon them into submission to ensure some action would follow. I suppose I was still in this mindset at the start of my seeing Alan. I still believed I would have to fight Alan so that I got the outcome I needed, in this case some therapy. One day, Alan decided to bring this up. He listened to me, paused, and said 'you know, you don't have to be a warrior in here.'

I really like those shoes, Alan

During one of the early sessions, I found myself moving off topic and complimenting Alan on his stylish leather shoes. I now know that I was looking for a respite after diving into some acutely painful memories. Alan simply nodded and said nothing, visibly eager to move off the topic and get back onto our original topic. I thought about this incident over the next week and during our next session, I told him how it made me feel. This led to a 30-minute discussion in which he apologised and took ownership of it, saying how he always found it hard to take compliments. Far from harming our partnership, the simple, humble and honest way he dealt with this incident brought us closer.

Moving chair

One day, during one session, I realised that at the start of each session, I was moving my chair forward very slightly – by maybe one inch. I asked Alan and he confirmed he too had noticed. Alan did not offer immediate interpretations but allowed me some space to understand the cause of it. In the course of the session, I was able to realise that by pulling my chair closer to him, I was subconsciously trying to block the way to the door and therefore stopping him from leaving out of social embarrassment, at my emotionally impoverished background. We spent the rest of the double session exploring this topic. He told me that whilst one reason might be the dominant cause of a behaviour, there are often several many others, all playing a part. 'People can feel more than one thing', and this is one of Alan's teachings that I use on a daily basis.

At the start of the next session, I still found myself unconsciously moving my chair forward, before immediately realising. I was confused. 'But Alan, we've covered this, why am I doing it still?' Alan explained that change takes time and encouraged me to be kind to myself. And sure enough, after a few sessions where the chair position was discussed, changed, reverted (I even spent a whole session sitting as far away from him as possible), I eventually got to a point where I was able to keep my chair back permanently.

A couple of years later we did revisit this period and had a laugh about it. I asked him 'God Alan, what must have you been thinking when you saw that?'. With his characteristic smile, he simply said that there were just some things to look at.

'Bollocks'

As the months went by, Alan and I began exploring even more areas of my life. Looking back, I can see that I was becoming comfortable with Alan. I was feeling at home in the therapy room, and tellingly I had started taking off my shoes before beginning to speak. In September 2011 James, François and I went to a much needed 2-week holiday in Turkey. I carried on with my weekly slot over the phone and during one session I started talking about my feelings towards the sea. I had as far as I could remember been terrified of the sea. 'The sea does not care about you, it could kill you without even knowing it. You are powerless when facing the sea.' Alan listened and paused. 'It does sound like you are talking about something else there.' I was truly not sure what he was talking about. 'Well, it does sound like you are talking about your mother.' I remember my reaction. 'Alan, with due respect, you are talking bollocks!' It was the first time I poo-pooed his interpretation. I thought it was such a facile therapy cliche. However, the information he had planted percolated in my mind and by the time of the very first session after the holiday, I could see he was right. Growing up I was always at the mercy of my mother's unpredictable mood and her outbursts of physical violence. After beating one of my brothers with a wooden clog, he needed seven stitches on his forehead. I heard my mother tell the doctor at A&E that my brother had fallen down the steps into a door. I was terrified that this could be me one day. And indeed, she had even once told me 'I got you into this world, I can take you out'.

One major breakthrough came when I recounted how my mother would often say after the divorce that she was both my mother and my father. Exploring this took up most of the session. Alan simply stated that this was impossible, and was an attempt at denying plain reality. She could only ever physically be my mother. Something in me changed that day, and I understood what Alan meant. My initial weariness and defensiveness disappeared and I could finally see that he was simply getting me to connect with the reality of my childhood.

Earlier, Alan had used the term 'absent dad' to describe my father. I did not understand, and had corrected him, stating that before the separation he was there in the house living with us. With characteristic patience Alan had simply said – 'Let's come back to this.' After the breakthrough, I got it. Again, he was not passing judgement, he was simply helping me to see things for what they were.

Alan made sure he spent a couple of sessions to explain that what I had gone through was not normal, and really it was abuse. Internally I had attributed this to all black families. But throughout this process, it always felt that we were side by side, metaphorically both looking into the well, rather than him being above me, and asking me to look into the well.

A few months later, I brought a CD player into the session and played him 'Snowflake' by Kate Bush. In this song Kate's son sings the role of a falling snowflake, that Kate promises to catch wherever it falls. It was a tearful session, and Alan gladly used this song as an entry point – I could explore what it would feel like to feel this level of support and love from one's mother.

Internalising Alan

Over the first year, the therapy process started earlier and earlier. On the day of therapy, I would find myself waking up more thoughtful, thinking things over that I would later unpack in session. Despite my request for 'homework', Alan would refuse to formally set any. Yet when sitting in front of him, it felt like I was receiving a lesson from a master or a sage, something that I could easily assimilate. Alan would always pause to consider things before speaking, nothing was ever said flippantly. My questions would usually be met with a 'well, let's look at this', followed by a careful exploration, done collaboratively.

Buffer time

At my request, Alan always gave me a 15-minute warning before the end of the session, to allow a gentle climbdown. But he had also been suggesting for a while to take a 'buffer' after therapy. This is a period of time to allow the mind to settle and rest before going out in the world again, and (in my case) resuming care duties for James. It took me a while to allow myself to do it – I felt James was in greater need. One week however, I bumped into Alan in the local Costa before our session. This triggered an honest conversation in session where Alan simply asked me what I wanted to do when bumping into him outside the session. He said some patients prefer not to acknowledge him, others do, and he was happy to do either. I was by that point very evangelical about therapy and Alan in particular (and still am!) and the idea to ignore Alan felt utterly wrong.

Classic Alan

I can hear Alan in my head on a weekly basis, dispensing what became one of his recurrent prompts. 'Marvin, do you really have time for this?' I have a very keen sense of justice, and whenever faced with people or companies doing the wrong thing, or getting away with a bad deed, my immediate instinct is to ensure they are held to account. Alan got me to think about this, and accept that there are limits to my time and energy. I also began to accept that it is not up to me alone to right all the world's wrong. Whenever I feel compelled to pursue a minor complaint, I hear Alan's question and reassess.

Alan becomes James's therapist

At the end of 2011, the relationship with James's original psychotherapist began to breakdown. Though it was never officially communicated, it felt like he was going through some personal problems of his own, and they had started to spill over into his work. François and I started talking about getting Alan to treat James too. For us it was really the obvious solution. We knew Alan and his great skills, and it would also allow a more joined up approach between the care work we delivered at home and the therapy Alan would dispense. We now know how unconventional this approach actually is, and how it goes against most clinical doctrine. In fact, much later we realised how difficult it is for a therapist to do well. The complex triangular dynamics, the potential for James to lose confidence in his therapist (as he now shared a therapist with his carer) are ever present. The CDS and Alan after a period of reflection agreed that after the Christmas break James would be treated by Alan as well. Alan would see James one-on-one twice a week and would run a weekly support therapy session with me.

Alan would discuss general themes of the sessions with James, whilst retaining his full trust. We still don't fully understand how Alan managed this setup so effortlessly. In my session I would contribute what was happening at home, and what we were working on with him. Alan would give advice on how to handle James's acting out, and support with any questions I had. Magically, Alan was on everyone's side. The first therapist James saw after Alan's death clearly could not manage this, and her relationship with both us and James broke down catastrophically. We realised that the clinical model that Alan provided to us was not something that all clinicians were able to do.

Bringing François into the support therapy

For a few months at the start of 2012, Alan had been telling me that he wanted to open the support therapy sessions to François. I must admit I was reluctant – I felt quite possessive of the relationship I had built with Alan over the last year or so. But eventually we arranged for the weekly sessions to become joint.

François's first experiences with Alan

Changing our family dynamics

The first area I remember Alan wanted to look at was about dynamics between James, Marvin and me. He was very clear that as well as caring for James, we were essentially reparenting him. And thus, we had to be aware of attempts by James to drive a wedge between us, and play us off against each other. So, we had to present a united front to him. We had to set boundaries and reassert the importance of our couple. We also had to harmonise our care, so that I would be a little bit like Marvin, and Marvin would be a little bit like me. Marvin's approach before therapy with Alan was to provide a total shielding to James from anything negative. Any trigger or negative experience felt catastrophic. I was more optimistic that James could overcome hurdles. In the immensely pressured and stressful context of James's early years in his recovery, this was often painted by Marvin as a lack of care or interest and I ended up almost convincing myself that this was the case. In one of the first joint sessions with Alan we dealt with this toxic divide. Alan simply pointed out that I clearly must care deeply about James, given all the sacrifices I had made in the previous 30 months. For the first time since we had started caring about James, there was someone independent, ready to support me and fight my corner. A huge load had lifted off my shoulders.

Still, a lot of work still had to be done. I was more hands off with James and also less likely to confront him if he acted out. Over time, we managed to bridge this gap. I remember using Alan's teachings to one day tell James that he was not talking to me with enough respect and that I was not there in his life to be used as a punching bag. It felt very empowering. On another occasion (much later), because he was not getting the response he wanted from Marvin, James turned to me. I gave the same response as Marvin, and he was clearly furious! The splitting of our couple, that he had managed to do so many times before, was no longer working.

I had little experience of therapy before meeting Alan and therefore some of his feats only became clear over time. But I still have admiration on how he managed to work with us all at the same time, and keep everyone's trust. We each felt Alan was 'our' therapist.

'Normalising'

Another strong theme in the first few years of the work was what he called 'normalising' things. It took a skilled therapist like him, sitting on the outside of our family unit, to undertake this process. Looking back, the three of us were under extreme pressures. Without really realising it, to compensate for James's truly appalling childhood abuse, Marvin and I wanted to protect him from any negative experience in the present. He was easily triggered in everyday life by things that would remind him of past trauma – a person with a tattoo, a severely obese woman, cursing on the TV. We did everything we could to remove risk of such triggers. For instance, entering a restaurant would require a quick scan of the customers, and selecting a table away from any trigger. We even stopped watching Downton Abbey when the plot included the rape of one of the characters (we only finished watching it eight years later, when James was living independently).

On the other hand, we wanted to fill his life with fun, uplifting experiences, that would, if not erase all the trauma, at least provide new positive memories alongside it. And frankly, we also welcomed these. Holidays, playground visits, elaborate picnics, horse riding experiences, trips to safari parks, all were organised for that purpose. At Christmas and birthdays, we were organising six presents for each of James's emotional personalities. But Alan clearly saw the imbalance building up. Our couple was suffering as James's needs became more important than any others. Marvin was exhausting himself, desperately aiming for perfection, and constantly; the underlying belief was that James would break down if confronted with more trauma. But as Alan got us to realise, it was also not healthy for James as he was not learning what real life is about. Alan spent a lot of therapy time on getting Marvin to accept that it was ok not to be perfect. He kept re-iterating how important it was to 'normalise' things. That meant treating each individual's needs as equally important, and allowing James to experience failure and the fact that his carers were human and therefore imperfect. A motto that he would repeat to all three was 'be kind to yourselves'. Marvin would use it whenever he was tempted to beat himself up about the quality of his care for James. Another related sentence that Alan would issue when Marvin was reaching for perfection was 'Marvin, it's good enough'.

The 'normalising' piece of work was accelerated by the fact that Alan now had access to both James and us, his carers, on a weekly basis. Yet, this took a long time to implement. For Marvin, the need to save James was rooted in his own childhood. Many times he had prayed that someone would come along and take him away from his hellish home life. For James, Marvin felt he was that saviour.

In the room where it happened

As we are writing this, we fear that we are not doing full justice to the talents of Alan as a therapist. We've both experienced a lot of eulogies that post-humously granted the deceased many qualities that they did not have in life. The opposite is true here: whatever words we can conjure will not cover the brilliance of Alan. He really was a virtuoso, a Mozart (or Rachmaninov if you prefer) of therapy. It looked deceivingly easy to us, yet the changes he effected were infinitely deep. There was an audible rhythm to Alan's therapy, which was conducted unseen. The melody was transfixing, and you awoke in the morning with its refrain clearly in your mind.

James once drew a picture of Alan, sitting in his therapy room cross legged, hiding a magic wand behind his back. And really it did capture how we also felt about him. His understanding of the human experience felt supernatural. When Alan died, it suddenly dawned on us how young he still was. In fact, Alan was Marvin's age, but his natural leadership and wisdom suggested a much older man. As someone else that knew him very accurately noted, we all wanted 'to be like Alan when we grew up', regardless of our age.

Alan's dedication to us was total, and he made us feel completely held. He had a natural flair and would assess each situation on a case-by-case basis, staying clear of rigid dogmas. Alan was happy for us to sit wherever in the room, and even conducted part of a session with James with him sitting upside down!

Alan's voice was quiet and gentle, but full of confidence and would draw you in. Never did he sound grandiose, arrogant or would make us feel like he alone held the knowledge. You really could not detect any misplaced ego in him. Many time we complemented him on the wonderful work he was doing with us and James, but he would invariably protest and say that it was us that were doing the work.

We think that compassion was a key ingredient in how successful Alan was. James told us early in his therapy how Alan had gained his trust by showing simple compassion when he was sharing details of his abuse. Instead of pre-senting an odd grimace as his previous therapist would do, Alan would gently shake his head and say 'gosh, that is awful'. It was simple but very powerful. We all firmly believed that Alan cared deeply about us and what we had gone through. On the rare occasions that we spoke to Alan on the telephone after the treatments ended Alan was always keen to ask how James was doing; it was clear that Alan was invested in James's ongoing well-being.

When it came to the weekly appointments, the start and end times would be firmly fixed. On the other hand, Alan was happy to support us on the phone on an ad hoc basis. For instance, Marvin spoke to him for about 45 minutes after his 15-year-old nephew committed suicide – showing both flexibility and humanity. If sessions had to be moved (as his work in Ireland with the An Garda Síochána would sometimes require), Alan would always give plenty of notice and usually offer an alternative slot that week. There was a strong feeling that Alan was providing a safe, dependable, warm environment. The image of a reinforced giant ostrich egg comes to mind as we write this, one where somehow time slowed down, and things can be looked at carefully, under the undivided gaze of a sympathetic mentor. In every session, it really felt like we were Alan's only patients.

Alan was secure enough to set limits on his 'hospitality' – he would offer a glass of water, but warm drinks were clearly off the menu! Overall nothing ever felt chaotic, or like he was overwhelmed by his own work. Alan was happy to admit his own mistakes when they rarely occurred, showing his humility and humanity, and reinforcing the confidence of his patients.

Above all, and maybe this is where Alan differs from other therapists we have come across, his therapy had a strong moral element to it – without ever sounding preachy. We would often ask him when faced with a difficult situation, what to tell James? His answer would always be 'what about just telling him the truth?'. And it was immediately obvious to us that this was of course the right course of action.

Alan was also able to speak up when he felt we were about to make a grave mistake. His sentence of choice would be in such situations 'I would think very carefully about doing this', which was really the strongest warning he would issue. But this would be really a last resort, his normal style being more Socratic by aiming to get us to the answer on our own. In fact, he told us he saw therapy as a space in which to think; and its main result as better thinking. Whenever we uncovered an unhealthy pattern, if we asked 'how do we stop making this mistake?', he would state: by being aware of it and practising good thinking. It was also a recurring theme with James and he taught us to ask James, whenever he acted out, 'what were you thinking at the time?'

Alan's death

We had spoken to Alan a couple of times after he stopped seeing us in 2014. In 2015 he was kind enough to try and mediate the rift between James's new therapist and the three of us. It was a relief to see him appearing healthy and in good spirits. It was therefore completely unexpected to hear in December 2016 from Dr Valerie Sinason that his cancer had returned and that he was likely to die in the coming weeks. We were shell-shocked. Sure enough the phone call came, only a few days later. Alan had died. It felt unreal. James was heart-broken and started wailing. We will always remember the voice of

Valerie repeating 'it's really rotten news, it's really rotten'. We were torn between our own grief and our duty of care towards James, who was deeply affected. We put our grieving process on hold, and focused on getting James through his turmoil.

A memorial service for Alan, held at the Freud Museum one year after his death, helped us to start processing his loss. Hearing from all manner of professionals, from therapists to social workers, whose lives were all touched by Alan, was amazing. It came as complete news to us that Alan was such a towering figure in the psychotherapy world. The creation of Respond, the groundbreaking work around disability, the training of the Gardaí back in Ireland, and simply how many people looked up to him and were deeply changed by his kind guidance – all of it was uplifting and bittersweet at the same time.

Alan's death was a tragedy, and no change of perspective can undo that. But we do feel privileged to have received some of his wisdom. Never has the saying 'may his memory be a blessing' made more sense. His kind advice still reverberates in our minds daily. As we re-read this piece, readying it for submission, his voice is there, saying gently: it's good enough.

Post Script

We wish to thank the following people, who along the years have made huge contributions to James' and our lives. We could not have done it without their help and benevolent attention.

Dr Valerie Sinason, for the invaluable help she has extended over the last ten years, and for being a beautiful, caring human being. Thanks for the cups of tea that always soothed Marvin's soul!

Cate Potter, who out of the goodness of her heart, was happy to support us 'pro bono', before the treatment package was approved. To this day, Cate still supports us.

Mark Renwick, for taking an interest in James' case and being compassionate and caring. A true role model for all psychiatric nurses!

Helena Bladon, for her weekly carer support sessions, which were a life line before Marvin's support therapy with Alan.

Epilogue

Valerie Sinason

Every year new research shows us that our ancestors of thousands of years ago were more skilled, relational and symbolic than we ever thought. Every year we learn more about the capacities of babies, including while still in the womb.

There is a longing in our adult species to feel "post-modern", the apex of civilisation and to consider that our newest trainings and understandings are the ultimate. Indeed, mental health professionals have allowed their training bodies to insist references need to be from the last five years only to prove we are up to date. Avoid Shakespeare, Confucius, Freud…

But all our work and research in this book comes from something precious, timeless and old. Old because Love is old yet timeless. Bowlby helped everyone by using the term "attachment", which does not carry baggage about sentimentality or corrupted toxic love. However, we need to return to the concept of professional love. It is literally as well as symbolically the heart of everything.

Love matters even more in work with those who have been emotionally wounded, stigmatised, excluded or falsely included. Love for our clients, our colleagues, our supervisors and supervisees and ourselves. Through that comes transformational change.

Something else is old yet also timeless. Look at most of the authors of these chapters and you find people who have been pioneers in this field for decades as well as working hard in the present tense. Pioneers in Ireland, the UK, Europe, Canada. We are all loyal to this field out of love and hold our arms out to welcome others to the IPD. We are holding the baby with disability to aid self-empowerment and growth. We are committed to ongoingness.

Our theories and findings have been accepted by government and trainings but the tragic reality of many wasted lives and units has not altered. There remains a fear of getting close to stigma, shame, trauma, difference. Despite the Olympic transformations we witness in our work there is a long way to go.

DOI: 10.4324/9781003646242-18

I have the privilege of being both a grandparent in this field and a daughter. My luminous father, the late Professor Stanley Segal OBE ensured the educational rights and inclusion of children with intellectual disability via his book *No Child Is Ineducable*. I have also had the privilege of teaching and being taught by almost all the fine writers and thinkers in this book.

So we are a timeless movement, us relational psychodynamic advocacy decolonial workers in the field of disability. Join us!

Index

For Product Safety Concerns and Information please contact our EU
representative GPSR@taylorandfrancis.com
Taylor & Francis Verlag GmbH, Kaufingerstraße 24, 80331 München, Germany

www.ingramcontent.com/pod-product-compliance
Lightning Source LLC
Chambersburg PA
CBHW050643280326
41932CB00015B/2761